T0093677

ENDEMIC

ENDEMIC

A POST-PANDEMIC PLAYBOOK

Monica Gandhi, M.D.

Mayo Clinic Press

MAYO CLINIC PRESS
200 First St. SW
Rochester, MN 55905
mcpress.mayoclinic.org

The information in this book is true and complete to the best of our knowledge. This book is intended as an informative guide for those wishing to learn more about health issues. It is not intended to replace, countermand, or conflict with advice given to you by your own physician. The ultimate decision concerning your care should be made between you and your doctor. Information in this book is offered with no guarantees. The author and publisher disclaim all liability in connection with the use of this book. The views expressed are the author's personal views, and do not necessarily reflect the policy or position of Mayo Clinic.

To stay informed about Mayo Clinic Press, please subscribe to our free e-newsletter at mcpress.mayoclinic.org or follow us on social media.

For bulk sales to employers, member groups, and health-related companies, contact Mayo Clinic at SpecialSalesMayoBooks@mayo.edu.

Proceeds from the sale of every book benefit important medical research and education at Mayo Clinic.

Cover design by Pete Garceau

Cataloging-in-Publication data is available from the Library of Congress.

ISBN: 978-1-945564-54-3 hardcover
ISBN: 978-1-945564-55-0 ebook

Printed in U.S.A.

First edition: 2023

This book is dedicated to my late husband, Dr. Rakesh K. Mishra, who battled cancer bravely for almost ten years and died three months before the COVID-19 pandemic. He was the most courageous, spiritual, vivacious, intelligent, and loving person I have ever known. It was truly my honor and joy to share part of my life and our children with this luminous being.

CONTENTS

ENDEMIC

Introduction

wanted to be an infectious diseases (ID) doctor since 1981, when I was twelve years old. The year was no coincidence; that was when AIDS was first described by the Centers for Disease Control and Prevention (CDC) in two devastating *Morbidity and Mortality Weekly Report*s discussing terrible opportunistic infections among gay men in San Francisco, New York City, Los Angeles, Miami, and Philadelphia.[1] Very soon thereafter, it became clear that HIV was an infection of disparities, preying upon poverty, social injustice, stigma, prejudice, and a lack of resources.

To fulfill this dream of working in ID, I went to medical school at Harvard and then to the University of California, San Francisco (UCSF) in 1996 for my medical residency and ID fellowship; I followed up with a Master's in Public Health from the University of California, Berkeley, specializing in epidemiology and biostatistics. Since then, my focus has been on HIV and disparities-based research at UCSF's public hospital. San Francisco was a natural place for me to work given that the city was the epicenter of the US HIV epidemic at the time.

I have had the privilege of treating people with HIV for more than twenty years now, working in and then directing a clinic that serves low-income, publicly insured patients in San Francisco (the Ward 86 HIV Clinic at San Francisco General Hospital). Over that time, my patients taught me everything I would need to know when the COVID-19 pandemic hit in early 2020. I responded by producing more than sixty-five op-ed pieces on COVID-19 in the mainstream press, making multiple podcast and media appearances, putting out social media posts, and now writing this book. My patients taught me how to champion biomedical advances to prevent and treat infectious disease (as we did with HIV); reminded me of the tenets of harm reduction and the need to take stigma, loneliness, and mental health effects into account when discussing the pandemic; and stressed activism, pragmatism, and resilience in a public health response. As one of my patients, who had children in the public schools in San Francisco (which were closed for a long time), kept saying to me throughout the pandemic: "Don't back down, Dr. Gandhi. We didn't back down with HIV. Let's get our kids back in school." I consider the work I did during COVID-19 to encourage school reopenings in the United States as both science-based— all the pieces I wrote referred to published or emerging data on COVID-19—and advocacy-based.[2] In the field of HIV, clinicians and researchers have always joined patients, advocates, and community-based organizations when it comes to activism based on data.

Based on history, I—and most other ID doctors—knew in the spring of 2020 that SARS-CoV-2 (the name of the virus that causes COVID) was not a pathogen that could be eradicated.[3] A knowledge of the history of infectious diseases told us that only one pathogen has ever been eradicated from humans worldwide: smallpox. (Rinderpest, a cattle virus, has been eradicated from cattle, but that was accomplished through mass execution of animals.) Smallpox was successfully eradicated worldwide in 1979, not only through the development of a vaccine but also because of some unique characteristics of that virus.[4] By contrast, SARS-CoV-2 has none of the features of smallpox (such as a lack of animal reservoirs)[5] that made it eradicable. That means we will always have to deal with COVID-19, much as we do with other non-eradicable respiratory pathogens, such as influenza and the viruses that cause the common cold.

When I first heard about HIV, I was living in Utah, where I was born and raised. A conservative state, Utah did not immediately incorporate education about this virus into our public school curriculum. The president of the United States at the time of the CDC's initial AIDS case series in the *Morbidity and Mortality Weekly Report,* Ronald Reagan, did not even acknowledge AIDS; indeed, President Reagan did not discuss AIDS until 1985, and there was a distinct feel from the administration that "Just Say No," the slogan that was a major part of the administration's anti–substance use initiatives, was also an easy way to control infectious diseases. Others pushed back, saying that merely being human predisposes us to being susceptible to infectious pathogens and that abstinence-only approaches were not appropriate public health responses to HIV.

When COVID-19 hit our planet in early 2020, I fully expected the same public health officials who had opposed an abstinence-only approach in attempting to control the spread of HIV to disagree with an eradication-based approach in attempting to control the spread of COVID-19 (because, of course, COVID-19 cannot be eradicated).[6] I expected them to say that we must do everything we can to control the spread of a pathogen like COVID-19 but that we must also take real-world conditions into account to minimize the harm caused by our interventions (harm reduction). To my surprise, many did not.

Instead, the political narrative in our country moved toward ignoring the harm of some of our efforts to control COVID-19, even when these interventions did not actually control the virus. Massive and prolonged school closures, indefinite postponement of medical care for other conditions, and keeping family members from seeing each other in hospitals and long-term care facilities during COVID-19 were the three main interventions that both caused harm and did not check the spread of COVID-19. Moreover, for a long time, the mainstream media did not effectively cover the damage from these ineffectual interventions; only in late 2022 did the media finally begin calling school closures a failed policy in that they caused harm to children without saving lives.[7] Going forward, as we codify the post-COVID-19 pandemic playbook, we have to acknowledge how to control the next pandemic without causing harm, using principles of *both* infection control and harm reduction, like we did for HIV.

In the United States, the first two years of COVID-19 resulted in poorer outcomes for racial and ethnic minorities, both from the virus and from the response to the virus in terms of workplace and school closures. This was very obvious in a city like San Francisco, which already had been grappling with vast disparities in wealth, as the poor bore the brunt of both the pandemic and the response to it.

My interest in studying disparities in HIV outcomes stemmed mainly from growing up in the United States as an Indian American. My family and I traveled from Utah to visit India when I was a child, and as an adult I've worked on HIV in both India and East

Africa. Witnessing outbreaks of infectious diseases in India and in poor communities in the United States, especially when those diseases were so easily controlled in rich communities, broke my heart. Inequities have always made low-income populations more susceptible to infectious diseases, including HIV and COVID-19, and I wanted desperately to combat these disparities.

Moreover, it is important to note that *responses* to infectious diseases also often disproportionately hurt the poor. To take one example from history, during the 1831 cholera epidemic in London, affluent residents could stay in their homes and have poor residents bring them food and water.[8] By using the less-affluent as a buffer, the response to this cholera outbreak deepened poverty in the parts of London most affected by the epidemic. This historical fact made me interested in taking a "resources before restrictions" approach to COVID-19—that is, providing people with the information and tools they need to stay safe, rather than imposing sweeping restrictions that have many negative consequences.[9]

Poverty has always made populations more susceptible to a host of pathogens and diseases. However, poverty has massively intensified worldwide as a result of COVID-19 and our response to it.[10] The number of children living in multidimensional poverty—with inadequate access to education, healthcare, housing, nutrition, sanitation, and clean water—increased by 150 million (to 1.2 billion) in 2020, and an additional 100 million children fell into poverty in 2021.[11] The need to reduce harm from our interventions when working to control new or existing pandemics is now obvious.

Furthermore, countries without universal healthcare, like the United States, fared more poorly in controlling disparities in health outcomes from COVID-19 than countries with national healthcare systems.[12] In my opinion, one of the most important lessons of this pandemic is the need for universal healthcare coverage and the obligation to recognize healthcare as a right, not a privilege.

Finally, both as an ID doctor working with people with HIV and as a brown woman in the United States, I am alert to stigma. When I was growing up, I was surprised that I would sometimes be judged for the color of my skin, which was an indisputable fact that I could not change. I was equally astounded that LGBTQ+ communities were judged for their sexuality and higher risk for certain infections, such as HIV, because of facts they could not change. In this spirit, I was disturbed when public health officials used stigmatizing terms to refer to people who contracted COVID-19, which is caused by a highly transmissible respiratory virus, when the very fact of being human made us all susceptible. I was surprised when some politicians and doctors said that those who remained unvaccinated for COVID-19 should not be treated should they fall ill. People were not "bad" or "COVidiots" if they contracted COVID-19; they were human. The role of public health is to educate people about how to stay safe from a virus, positively motivate the public to behave in health-promoting ways, and provide resources for such behaviors. There is absolutely no place for stigma, judgment, and a shame-based approach in public health when dealing with an infectious pathogen.

To be able to begin to "live with the virus," we had to wait until we got an effective COVID-19 vaccine and developed therapeutic agents to control the virus in populations more at risk of a severe breakthrough infection (an infection in someone who's been vaccinated). We also had to work on the entire world having access to the biomedical advances in the control and treatment of COVID-19. When I was growing up, I couldn't think of a topic more grounded in social justice and activism than HIV, which in the 2000s was disproportionately ravaging populations in sub-Saharan Africa even as highly effective antiretroviral medications were being developed and rolled out for the United States and Europe. HIV researchers and clinicians, along with HIV-affected communities, took to the streets to fight this injustice. This experience with HIV led to my interest in global and domestic vaccine and therapeutic equity for COVID-19, which I wrote about in multiple forums.[13] Distributing biomedical advances for any pathogen equitably across the world needs to be a major part of any pandemic response.

Even with the vaccines and effective therapeutics for COVID-19 that had been developed, the polarization of the COVID-19 response continued worldwide well into 2022, mainly in China (which maintained a lockdown approach until December 2022, despite difficulties in the country as a result) and the United States (where different states took different approaches, largely along political lines). By September 2022, the World Health Organization (WHO) declared that the end of the pandemic was in sight, but correctly warned the world that we would continue to need ongoing vaccination and therapeutics in the face of this non-eradicable virus.[14] However, by this time, the barrage of fear-based messaging to encourage compliance with public health measures, along with a failure to reassure the public of the power of our technical advances to fight the virus (a failure most pronounced in the United States), had led to widespread negative mental health effects in the population.[15] Also that September, the US Preventive Services Task Force made the historic decision to recommend screening for anxiety for all adults under sixty-five, even those who appeared asymptomatic, given the increased prevalence of adverse mental health conditions in the United States.[16]

On a personal note, my husband, the father of my two children, died in November 2019 (three months before the pandemic) after battling cancer for almost a decade. I am no stranger to anxiety regarding illness. This terrible and indisputable fact of my life heightened my awareness of how the public health response to COVID-19 favored those with the privilege of having two parents around in the face of prolonged school closures or having an intact family when telling someone to "just say no" to seeking comfort outside their immediate circle. Finally, the response to COVID ignored the mental health effects of stigmatizing people for craving human companionship.

Our children and I were unable to lay my dearly beloved husband to rest in the Ganges River in India until the post-pandemic period of the summer of 2022. I loved my husband beyond measure and really thank him for the love he gave me and our two sons through his courageous, spiritual, and epic battle against mortality. He gave me everything; I give the world my impressions of COVID-19 and, I hope, a way forward for the next pandemic as we face a world at risk for the spread of more pathogens due to our treatment of animals, climate change, a global loss of trust in public health officials, and setbacks in both routine childhood vaccinations and vaccine confidence.[17]

This book tries to take the hard-won lessons from the response of HIV and apply them to evaluating the COVID-19 response so that we can develop a post-pandemic playbook to inform our response to the next pandemic. We can learn, from HIV and now COVID-19, about compassion, reason, biomedical advances, transparency, equitable access, global development, and the importance of acknowledging uncertainty.[18]

CHAPTER 1

HIV as Prophet and Teacher for COVID-19

The last great infectious disease pandemic prior to COVID-19 was HIV. HIV can be a prophet and teacher for COVID-19 in a way that we are just beginning to understand. The polarization, politicization, and divisiveness around HIV were mirrored during the COVID-19 pandemic, but we could have harnessed many lessons from HIV to deal with COVID-19: lessons around the importance of biomedical interventions to get back to "normal life" and lessons around harm reduction.[1] I think there are three reasons we did not learn these lessons: politics, messaging to increase compliance, and fear.

Politics. When AIDS battered the United States in the early 1980s, as we've seen, President Ronald Reagan at first refused to discuss HIV at all. Then, when he did address it, he advanced an abstinence-only approach to combat the virus. Understanding that neither silence nor abstinence would be effective, public health officials took on the task of supplying information and promoting harm-reduction strategies, both of which put them in opposition to the president.[2] This took on a political cast, because Reagan was coming from the right and public health officials tend to lean left (as do I). Forty years later, when COVID-19 hit, in the initial stages of the pandemic, President Donald Trump didn't treat it as the serious threat it was.[3] To counter this (and also in some cases for political reasons), public health and mainstream messaging greatly emphasized the danger posed by SARS-CoV-2. As a result, much media coverage was fear-based, even if there was good news, as when the vaccines came out.[4] The *New York Times* noted in 2021 that the US media tended to present bad news about COVID, and sometimes the information they were presenting wasn't even fact-based. In this respect, the United States was an outlier—in 2020, about 87 percent of COVID coverage in national US media was negative, but negative coverage in international media was only 51 percent and in scientific journals 64 percent.[5] Public health officials in the United States did not extol the vaccines as a way back to normal life, as officials in other countries did, nor did they routinely criticize the effects of prolonged school closures. In their reporting, the US progressive press tended to follow left-leaning public health officials.

For instance, I was asked to discuss COVID-19 on *Democracy Now* several times, and in May 2021, during the short window in which the CDC said the vaccinated need not mask, I commented that any push to continue mask-wearing even after vaccination might give the public the idea that vaccines do not work. However, my view was not considered part of the progressive narrative at the time, and so it never gained traction in those circles or in the mainstream media. In the Scandinavian countries, by contrast, which as a whole are more left-leaning but less polarized, vaccines were universally agreed upon as the way to resume normal life.[6]

Messaging to Increase Compliance. While there was initially some panic about HIV among the general population, we quickly learned that it is usually restricted to those at risk of a sexually transmitted or blood-borne pathogen. By contrast, everyone is susceptible to a highly transmissible respiratory virus like SARS-CoV-2; this led to widespread fear of the virus, which was reflected in the media. Here too, though, we soon came to see that some people were at greater risk of serious consequences than others, but this sober, data-based approach didn't make it into general coverage of the pandemic. Moreover, during the pandemic, it seems likely that in some cases a fear-based narrative was deliberately employed in order to ensure that the public complied with recommended public health measures.[7] However, there had already been numerous studies done in the context of HIV showing that fear-based messaging and an emphasis on abstinence were not nearly as effective as providing people with the information and tools they needed to stay safe from a pathogen (the "resources before restrictions" approach).[8] In short, people stay safer from infection when we give them empowering tools and information, rather than telling them to "just say no."

Fear. Fear sells papers and generates interest in online journalism—think "clickbait"—but it can lead to stress and anxiety.[9] Our job in medicine is to reassure, not to frighten unnecessarily. When treatments came along for HIV, we told our patients that this meant their lives would be normal, that they should know that we had them covered in terms of combating the immunosuppressing effects of HIV with medications. When pre-exposure prophylaxis (PrEP) for HIV came along, we told patients that, between the treatments and PrEP, condom use was not necessary during sex. We reassured people and provided calm and life-normalizing advice. Somehow, though, in the United States, the development of COVID-19 vaccines didn't seem to unlock the door to normal life as it did in other countries. Moreover, the fear-based media reporting of COVID continued in the United States for quite some time after the international press had ceased using this approach; for example, when it came to studies of long COVID (now also known as post-acute sequelae of SARS-CoV-2, or PASC), as late as October 2022 the US media gave prominent attention to flawed studies (those with low response rates, without adequate controls, and without any accounting for vaccination status).[10]

———

Let's delve a little deeper into the history of HIV to see how it could have served as a teacher for our response to COVID-19.

HIV/AIDS was first noted by the CDC on June 5, 1981, in a landmark *Morbidity and Mortality Weekly Report*.[11] The descriptions of unusual, serious infections that affected the eyes, skin, lungs, brain, and gastrointestinal tract—mainly in young gay men in San Francisco, Miami, New York City, Philadelphia, and Los Angeles—shook the world. These were infections that had previously been seen only in patients with profound immunosuppression from other causes and were often fatal. The human immunodeficiency virus (HIV) was identified as the etiologic agent behind acquired immunodeficiency syndrome (AIDS) by 1983, and the next decade and a half—until effective therapeutics were developed—were both heartbreaking and profoundly polarizing in the United States and around the world.[12]

Due to the stigmatization of the LGBTQ+ community in the United States, as noted, President Ronald Reagan did not mention AIDS at the time the infection was first described; it would take him four more years, until he was asked by a reporter about it in 1985, to even utter the word.[13] Although public health officials at first counseled that gay men should completely abstain from sex and tried to control gay male sexual activity by closing bathhouses and attempting to ban "bad" sex, it was quickly recognized that stigmatization and shaming were bad public health policy.[14] In fact, the more the federal government under President Reagan ignored HIV at first and then recommended an abstinence-only approach, the more the public health and infectious diseases community turned toward harm reduction as a more effective strategy for controlling transmission.[15]

As discussed before, this concept of harm reduction in infectious diseases stems from the HIV epidemic and revolves around the concept that public health recommendations to minimize the impact of a pathogen must also consider the other needs of affected individuals and communities. Harm reduction is the substratum of how we message about HIV risk and does not usually entail telling individuals to be abstinent but rather encourages them to use tools (initially condoms, and now pre-exposure prophylaxis and treatment) to minimize risk.[16] In the field of substance use and addiction, harm reduction has become a mainstay of public health management, standing in contrast to Nancy Reagan's "Just Say No" campaign against substance use, which was criticized by the public health community as being too simplistic.[17] Harm reduction aims to minimize the risk of exposure to pathogens from needles by providing clean needles and educating people on why using them is a good idea; it also seeks to provide counseling on reducing the negative consequences of drug use without requiring abstinence.[18]

At this point in the HIV response, we have highly effective antiretroviral therapies to control the disease, allowing individuals carrying the virus to live a normal and healthy life.[19] We have tools such as PrEP and treatment to serve as prevention (undetectable levels of the virus in an individual means they can't transmit the infection, hence the slogan "Undetectable Equals Untransmittable"). As a result, the risk of HIV infection from sex is so low that counseling condom use is no longer necessary for both same-sex and heterosexual partnerships.[20] But as we discussed in the introduction, the world did not provide equitable access to HIV therapies for millions of individuals living with HIV in poor countries until more than a decade after they were developed, adding to the tragedy and injustice of the infection (something we would see happen again with COVID-19 vaccines and therapeutics).[21] And even now, despite having the tools, we have a long way to go to end the HIV epidemic, as public attention and funding were flagging even before COVID-19 resulted in setbacks to the HIV response during and after the emergency phase of the pandemic.[22]

COVID-19 led to major backsliding in the HIV response. As of 2021, there were 38.4 million people living with HIV around the world; there were 650,000 deaths from HIV/AIDS and 1.5 million new infections in that same year, with a total of 40.1 million deaths since the beginning of the HIV pandemic. The statistics are particularly disturbing for young women. Every week in 2021, around 4,900 young women between ages fifteen and twenty-four became infected with HIV across the globe (that is a new infection every two minutes). In fact, in sub-Saharan Africa, six in seven new HIV infections among adolescents between the ages of fifteen and nineteen were among girls; prolonged school closures through the COVID-19 pandemic likely contributed to this disproportionate impact.[23] HIV is still a pandemic, mainly because the prevention and treatment tools have not been equitably applied worldwide. Plus, we still need an effective HIV vaccine, although very exciting trials are now underway to study mRNA vaccines for HIV infection, an advance informed by COVID-19 vaccine development.[24]

So, what happened with COVID-19 and our response in the United States? Chapters 2 and 3 describe the virus, discuss the vaccines and treatments that have been developed, and discuss how we have moved from the pandemic, a period in which the virus spread quickly and widely, with cases and then hospitalizations skyrocketing day after day, into a stage in which the virus is endemic—it is now consistently present, but rates of severe disease have greatly diminished.[25] COVID will now be monitored like the flu, which becomes more prevalent in different places at different times. But, before that evolution, the polarization and divisiveness around how to manage the pandemic were fierce.

What became clear early on is that SARS-CoV-2, unlike smallpox, is not a virus that can ever be completely eradicated.[26] Therefore, we knew that we needed to develop vaccines and therapeutics for this virus as soon as possible in order to get to a stage of control, in which we live with the non-eradicable infection by always applying tools to keep the rates of severe disease as low as possible.

The discipline of infectious diseases has strict definitions when it comes to describing levels of containment for a communicable disease.[27] "Control" means that a disease has been brought down to low levels of circulation with the help of public health interventions such as vaccines and therapeutics. "Elimination" means the incidence of disease has been reduced in a certain geographical region to zero. "Eradication" means the incidence of the disease worldwide has been reduced to zero.

Smallpox was successfully eradicated worldwide in 1979, not only because of the vaccine but also because of some unique characteristics of the virus.[28] It lacked an animal reservoir (that is, it did not occur in animals, from which it could spread to humans). It had clear pathogenic features that made it easy to quickly recognize in sufferers by its clinical signs and symptoms, such as the pox-like rash. It had a short period of infectiousness. And getting infected conferred natural immunity for life.

Measles is an example of a disease that can never be eradicated; this highly transmissible respiratory virus came under control after a vaccine was developed in 1963, and in regions where a large proportion of the population is vaccinated (as in the United States), it has technically been eliminated, although occasional outbreaks still occur. These outbreaks occur in areas of low vaccination, including in the wake of the COVID-19 pandemic—missed measles vaccinations, for example, led to more than 700 deaths among unvaccinated children in Zimbabwe in August 2022.[29]

The 1918 influenza pandemic was the deadliest pandemic in history, partially because we did not have an effective influenza vaccine until 1942; therefore, that disease came under control and became endemic only once the strain evolved to become less virulent and immunity in the population rose because of natural infection.[30]

SARS-CoV-2 has features that make it impossible to eradicate, including its high level of transmissibility, the ease with which its

symptoms can be mistaken for other common respiratory infections, and the ability of the virus to be transmitted even before
symptoms develop. Finally, the main reason that COVID-19 cannot be eradicated is that at least twenty-nine species of animals can
harbor the virus.[31] (One of these was recognized as early as April
2020, when COVID-19 was identified in big cats in a New York
zoo.) Viruses with this many animal reservoirs have never been
eradicated.

After initial lockdowns around the world, we used non-pharmaceutical interventions such as testing, contact tracing, face masks,
ventilation, and distancing to keep transmission as low as possible
while awaiting a vaccine.[32] And, in fact, the first emergency use authorization for a highly effective vaccine in the United States came
on December 11, 2020, just nine months after the World Health
Organization declared COVID-19 a pandemic.[33] But in our zeal to
get to COVID-zero—a strategy that by 2021 had been abandoned
by all countries but China—we seemed to forget the principles of
harm reduction along the way. Harm reduction would say that we
need to minimize the effects of COVID-19 while also not hurting
other aspects of public health, like mental health, education (which
is directly linked to future health outcomes), management of other
medical conditions, and trust in governments.[34]

For example, in the United States (unlike in the United Kingdom and Europe), we closed and then disrupted schools for extended
periods, longer in states led by Democrats than Republicans.[35] California was the last of the states to reopen schools after the initial
lockdowns, despite businesses and other parts of society being open.
This was a tragic mistake with potentially long-term consequences.

UNICEF stated in October 2020 that "schools must be the last places to close and the first to reopen."[36] Europe and the UK opened schools as soon as possible after shutting down. However, despite prolonged school closures not being part of prior pandemic playbooks, we in the United States kept ours closed or disrupted (often along party lines) for far longer than needed.[37]

In December 2021, a year after vaccines for COVID-19 were available in the US, the surgeon general of the United States declared a mental health crisis among US children and adolescents—a crisis that impacted groups disparately due to the existing systemic fissures of class and race.[38] And in May 2022, researchers at Harvard reported that pandemic academic learning loss was greatest in high-poverty school districts where learning was kept remote for longer.[39] The report predicted that the academic learning loss (as well as the negative social and emotional effects) suffered by mainly racial- and ethnic-minority children could have long-term consequences for occupational achievement unless we undertake a course correction. Plunging test scores reported in August 2022 portend a long road ahead for educational recovery in the United States.[40] Given that COVID-19 is a disease with a marked age stratification of risk (that is, children are at much less risk for severe disease than people at the other end of the age spectrum), the prolonged school closures in many of our states were not consistent with principles of harm reduction.[41]

I think there were two other major aspects of the US response to COVID-19 that were not consistent with the principles of harm reduction. One was the failure to allow family members to visit loved ones in hospitals or long-term care facilities, leading some states to pass laws in April 2022 that this fundamental aspect of being human can never be restricted again, even during outbreaks.[42] The other was that many states took a fear-based and not facts-based approach to managing COVID-19, which elevated anxiety and led many individuals to avoid medical care for their other important medical needs during the time of the pandemic.[43] As a result, we saw deaths from preventable causes, such as drug overdoses, alcohol use, and other chronic medical conditions (e.g., cancer, cardiovascular disease, strokes, diabetes), rise across the country.[44] Anxiety, disruption of access to healthcare facilities, prolonged periods of isolation, and economic uncertainty during our COVID response all took a serious toll on public health.

As discussed previously, when they're applied to disease prevention, the principles of harm reduction mean we should advise individuals how to mitigate the risk of infection within the greater human context of needs, including both economic and social needs. Harm reduction and abstinence do, in fact, have the same goal in the end: to reduce the overall impact of the infection.

Other mistakes stemming from the fear-based approach we took included not providing resources to help those most vulnerable to exposure with isolation and testing; failing to recognize how important universal healthcare is to helping reduce disparities in COVID-19 outcomes in countries like the United States; and stigmatizing people who contracted COVID-19 as "not following the rules."[45] With COVID-19 and the subsequent outbreak of monkeypox, public health authorities in the United States took a very different approach to stigmatizing messaging and harm reduction than they did with HIV.[46] Public health messaging around monkeypox (renamed Mpox) in the United States was much more aligned with principles of harm reduction and compassion. That was especially disconcerting in terms of COVID-19 messaging, given that we'd already seen how antithetical stigma and shame are to improving public health.[47]

As noted, our eventually largely successful response to HIV stressed minimizing transmission of the infection and minimizing the consequences of disease while simultaneously taking the other needs of individuals and communities into account. It's interesting that in the United States, the harm-reduction approach to HIV was mainly a progressive position, but during COVID-19, progressives and left-leaning mainstream media seemed to take a more abstinence-based, fear-based, and restriction-based approach to COVID-19. I am "left of left" in my political leanings, as evidenced by my voting and donation records, but I did not understand the position that many Democratic-led states took toward prolonged school closures and disruptions, while the Republican-led states typically worked harder to reopen schools. Moreover, I am aware of how important early education for girls is for their empowerment later in life (I coedited a book on women's empowerment and global health in 2016), and I knew the negative impact that closing schools would have on health outcomes among girls globally.[48]

I live in California, which had the longest public school closures of any state in the country (although most private schools were open, which deepened preexisting disparities). California was last among the fifty states in terms of in-person learning days during the pandemic; its neighbor just to the north, Oregon, was forty-ninth out of fifty.[49] Although California had not released its K–12 public school test scores for 2022 as of this writing, Oregon had, and the data highlighted disturbing inequities, with historically underserved student groups faring worst in terms of learning and predicted future occupational opportunity losses.[50]

Mixing politics with public health and failing to grasp the impact on the poor of draconian measures to prevent the spread of COVID-19 had social consequences.[51] In May 2021, a Pew poll showed that about half of Americans trusted the CDC; by January 2022, a Hart poll found that only 44 percent of Americans trusted the CDC; by March 2022, a Gallup poll put the level of trust at 32 percent.[52] We are now seeing the untoward effects of that mistrust, which is impacting uptake of vaccines for COVID and, more recently, other vaccine-preventable diseases, including influenza, measles, and polio.[53] The CDC announced a major reorganization in August 2022, citing missteps in the COVID pandemic response, to combat this erosion of trust in the premier American public health agency.[54]

The effects of fear-based messaging were very evident in California and especially San Francisco, which took one of the strictest lockdown approaches in the country. I saw patients with HIV throughout the pandemic, and the fear was very palpable early on, as patients would not come in for life-extending care for their HIV, cardiovascular disease, or cancer due to anxiety about contracting COVID-19 from the healthcare system. I had a patient who absolutely refused to come in when experiencing new shortness of breath, which ended up being severe congestive heart failure; it caused damage that could have been prevented with earlier treatment. Similarly, many healthcare systems closed their doors to all non-emergency in-person care.

At least 40 percent of the patients in Ward 86, the publicly funded HIV clinic for which I have served as medical director since 2014, have histories of substance use; some of them are in remission, but relapse was common during the loneliness and isolation of COVID-19. Overdose deaths in San Francisco skyrocketed during the pandemic and killed three times as many people in the city as the virus did.[55] We were fortunate at our large HIV clinic in San Francisco not to have had much severe disease from COVID-19, but the overdose deaths were frequent. In the city of San Francisco, seven people living with HIV died of COVID-19 in 2020 and 2021 combined, with 286 deaths total among those with HIV in 2020 (with the death statistics for 2021 not yet released).[56]

I have many patients at Ward 86 who suffered profoundly from loneliness and isolation during the COVID-19 pandemic. One white gay man in his sixties told me that this time felt like the early 1980s with HIV, except that instead of being told not to have sex, he was told "not to breathe around others." During one visit I asked a white bisexual man in his fifties about noisy neighbors he'd previously mentioned to me, but this time he hung his head and said, "They're dead. They're both dead from an overdose, and I miss the noise." A Black transgender woman in her forties broke up with her long-term boyfriend, as she "didn't know what he was doing with whom"—not in terms of sexual relationships but in terms of gathering indoors. A Latina cisgender woman in her late fifties was so sad when she was told not to see her daughter, son, and grandchildren that she started drinking alcohol heavily again and was hospitalized with alcohol-related complications. A young Latino bisexual man in his thirties contemplated suicide due to social isolation and finally moved to a state where he felt that laxer COVID-19 restrictions "allowed me to be more free to be me." In September 2022, an African American cisgender woman in her late sixties who had already received four doses of COVID-19 vaccine broke down in my office, saying she had not seen her mother and sister (who lived across the street) since the beginning of the pandemic. I asked if she would go see them—and bridge the chasm of loneliness she had experienced due to fear—if I ordered dinner for three to be delivered to her mother's house. That made her laugh, and she joked that "bribery was the only thing that would do it." Still, she reported back to me the next day that she loved seeing her family again.

SARS-CoV-2 is a deadly virus, but shaming people for craving human companionship is not consistent with the principles of harm reduction in combating infection. Before vaccines became available, my advice to my patients was to use non-pharmaceutical forms of protection (masking, ventilation, distancing) to see those they cared about.[57] After the vaccines were released, I tried to provide reassurance about how powerful they were at protecting against severe disease, even among the immunocompromised.[58]

Indeed, after the vaccines became widely available in the spring of 2021, I think we should have messaged more optimism instead of doom and gloom.[59] I believe the CDC was trying to motivate people to get vaccinated by saying in May 2021 that those who had been vaccinated were no longer required to wear masks. I agreed with this decision, mostly because I thought the prospect of returning to normal life would push vaccine uptake.[60] A study in the *Journal of Community Health* published in October 2021 asked those who were still hesitant to take a vaccine what would motivate them to get vaccinated. The most common theme was a desire to protect themselves from severe disease, and the second most common theme focused on a return to normal life, with the ability to stop wearing a mask a frequently noted feature.[61]

However, breakthrough infections (though typically mild) became more frequent with the delta variant wave. A SARS-CoV-2 outbreak in Provincetown, Massachusetts, led the CDC to recommend in July 2021 that everyone mask again, and that may have served to demotivate people from getting the vaccine.[62] This seemed to be a turning point in terms of trust of the CDC around public health messaging.[63] Paradoxically, the Provincetown outbreak, rather than being a clear signal that we all needed to mask up again, might better have been interpreted as a demonstration of the power of the vaccines to prevent severe disease when exposure is high. Briefly, a large LGBTQ+ gathering occurs in Provincetown each summer, and in the summer of 2021 everyone was in a celebratory mood, since the vaccines had been rolled out and many in the United States felt we were emerging from a difficult pandemic. However, with situations of very close contact among unmasked people in poorly ventilated conditions (such as in nightclubs), an outbreak of mild COVID cases occurred. There were a total of 469 cases, with three-quarters of them among vaccinated individuals. But the good news was that there was very little severe disease; there were only four hospitalizations and no deaths among the vaccinated.[64]

The failure at this point in the pandemic to promote how suc-cessful the vaccines were at preventing what we dreaded most about COVID-19—its ability to cause severe disease—may have been the greatest reason for the subsequent loss of trust in public health au-thorities and vaccines in the United States.[65] Vaccines are a much more effective tool than masks at preventing severe disease from SARS-CoV-2. If vaccines weren't going to return us to normal life, what would? In early September 2021 I tweeted, "The messaging over the last month in the U.S. has basically served to terrify the vaccinated and make unvaccinated eligible adults doubt the effec-tiveness of the vaccines." This tweet got more likes and retweets than any other I had put out; the *New York Times* even quoted it when explaining a few days later how the Provincetown outbreak actually showed that the vaccines were a success.[66] I truly do believe that the public health messaging in the United States around this time, which failed to take into account that vaccines were highly effective in preventing severe disease, led to less vaccine uptake and a lot of statements on social media to the effect that "vaccines don't work." The messaging in the United States during the delta variant surge contrasted sharply with that seen in highly vaccinated regions in northern Europe and in Singapore, where the fact that a rise in cases did not come with a parallel surge in hospitalizations was hailed as a vaccine success.[67] Indeed, during the delta variant surge, in recognition that mild infections would continue but that vac-cines prevented severe disease so effectively, Singapore decided to report only COVID hospitalizations, not total cases, to the public to minimize fear-based messaging.[68]

In highly vaccinated San Francisco, the delta variant led to increased cases but not hospitalizations, since vaccines decouple infections from severe disease.[69] And across the United States, vaccination rates were inversely related to hospitalizations due to the delta variant.[70] However, our failure in the summer of 2021 to message optimism regarding the vaccines' ability to prevent severe disease may have led to more negative mental health effects among the population, especially in those who had been so eager to receive the vaccine.[71] I wrote op-eds around that time on the power of cellular immunity, generated by the vaccines, to protect us against severe disease, and received hundreds of emails from people around the country who felt reassured by this optimism, which seemed to be missing from the media coverage.[72] One wrote, "It was only due to this compassionate, rational perspective that [my mother] started to see her grandson again. Otherwise, she remained fearful, as a triple vaccinated woman who is in good health. . . . You cannot imagine her isolation otherwise." A physician wrote, "Over the past year, I had become very depressed . . . after always being a positive person. . . . [M]uch of that changed the day I heard one of your podcasts. . . . [T]he constant reiteration of clinical, translational, and real-world data has been a breath of fresh air from the constant negativity reported in the media." In the United States, fear-based messaging has been so extreme that we seemed unable to see the light at the end of the tunnel even two years after the vaccines became widely available.[73] Would public health officials ever be able to regain people's trust?

CHAPTER 2

COVID-19

How It Spread, Whom It Affects
Most, and How It Causes Disease

The history of pandemics worldwide has always shown a disproportionate impact on the poor, with "intersecting social and economic inequalities" making the impact of the infection (*and* pandemic policies, in the case of COVID-19) worse in marginalized communities.[1] The COVID-19 pandemic was unusual in sparing children, as many other infectious diseases have a significant effect on both the very young and the very old. For instance, unvaccinated children are at highest risk of death from measles during outbreaks, as were the elderly prior to the availability of the measles vaccine.[2] Polio most adversely affects children under five years of age.[3] Respiratory syncytial virus (RSV)—which was very active in the winter of 2022—affects the very young and the elderly.[4] Seasonal influenza affects the very young and elderly most severely, although the 1918 influenza pandemic was unusual in targeting healthy young adults.[5] We knew early on in the COVID-19 pandemic (even in February 2020, from data coming out of Wuhan, China, and covered by mainstream progressive media) that this novel coronavirus mostly spared young children.[6] Nonetheless, the United States (unlike the United Kingdom or European countries) failed to take the disease's profound age gradient into account when making recommendations for the public and schools, which led to polarization and discord in our response.

A BRIEF HISTORY OF COVID-19

On December 31, 2019, the World Health Organization was informed of a cluster of cases of pneumonia of unknown etiology in Wuhan, a city in China's Hubei Province.[7] By January 7, 2020, a novel coronavirus (named severe acute respiratory syndrome coronavirus–2, or SARS-CoV-2) was identified in samples obtained from these patients, whose disease was labeled coronavirus 2019 (COVID-19).[8] Coronaviruses are RNA viruses (meaning they have RNA, rather than DNA, as their genetic material), and such viruses can infect humans, mammals, and birds, although most human coronaviruses (HCoVs) usually only cause the common cold in humans. Indeed, four circulating coronaviruses (HCoV-OC43, HCoV-229E, HCoV-NL63, and HCoV-HKU1) are responsible for 15–30 percent of all common colds in the population.[9] However, coronaviruses can cause severe disease, with SARS-CoV-2 the third or perhaps fourth example of a coronavirus causing severe pneumonias.

The first such coronavirus may have been HCoV-OC43.[10] Various reports now indicate that HCoV-OC43 may have been the virus behind the severe "Russian influenza" outbreak in Europe in 1889–1894, as demonstrated by sequencing studies of that virus that were recently performed.[11] The "Russian flu," which was a worldwide pandemic for those five years, is considered the first pandemic of the industrial era.[12] The outbreak started in the Russian Empire before spreading to Europe and the rest of the world. The virus was very contagious and had a relatively low case fatality rate (0.10–0.28 percent) compared to COVID-19, with an initial case fatality rate of 1.5–10 percent.[13] Nonetheless, the virus causing the "Russian flu" is estimated to have caused 1 million deaths worldwide. The genetic similarity between HCoV-OC43 and a bovine coronavirus that was causing disease among cattle in Europe at the same time makes it increasingly likely that this virus was the cause of this pandemic. If this is true, HCoV-OC43 would have been the first known example of a coronavirus causing severe disease in human populations. Over time, increasing immunity to the virus across the planet and the virus's evolution to a less virulent strain led to OC-43 becoming a mild endemic virus thereafter.[14]

The second time in recent human history that a coronavirus caused severe pneumonias—and the first pandemic of the twenty-first century—was the SARS pandemic.[15] In late 2002, a cluster of unexplained pneumonias emerged in Foshan, Guangdong Province, China. The disease, which was later identified as being caused by a novel coronavirus, was named severe acute respiratory syndrome (SARS); it spread to other countries and was labeled a pandemic by the World Health Organization in March 2003. The pandemic subsided after about nine months of circulation, with 8,096 cases and 774 deaths having been reported, giving the infection a mortality rate of approximately 10 percent.[16] SARS mainly spread from individuals with active symptoms. The virus originated from the horseshoe bat, went through a catlike mammal called the palm civet, and then entered human populations.[17]

The second time a coronavirus caused severe disease this century was during the MERS pandemic. Middle East respiratory syndrome (MERS) was first identified as a coronavirus-caused pneumonia in 2012 in Saudi Arabia; so far, all cases of MERS have been linked through travel to, or residence in, countries in and near the Arabian Peninsula. As of March 2022, there have been 2,589 confirmed cases with 893 associated deaths, giving this infection a case fatality rate of 34.5 percent.[18] The origin of this virus is also thought to be bats, and the virus likely passed through the dromedary and then was transmitted to humans.[19]

The most serious, widespread pandemic from a coronavirus is the COVID-19 pandemic, the seventh coronavirus identified as infecting humans. Although the precise source of the COVID-19 pandemic is uncertain, data suggests that the virus originated in bats and perhaps passed from animals to humans in the Wuhan wet market.[20] However, the animal intermediary has not yet been identified as of this writing, and in June 2022 the World Health Organization called for more investigation into biosafety in laboratories studying coronaviruses.[21]

THE EPIDEMIOLOGY OF COVID-19

Despite aggressive mitigation strategies, the infection rapidly spread, and on March 11, 2020, the WHO declared COVID-19 a global pandemic. Cases have occurred in every country. By November 2022, 6.6 million deaths from COVID-19 had been recorded, though that figure likely underreports the true number.[22] Moreover, there have been as many as 12 million excess deaths—that is, 12 million more deaths than would have been expected under normal conditions—as a result of medical problems not cared for adequately during the pandemic (including cardiovascular disease, cancer, strokes, and other infectious diseases) as well as from other indirect consequences of the pandemic.[23] At over 1 million COVID-19 deaths as of November 2022, the United States has had the highest absolute number and the second-highest number of deaths per capita from COVID-19 in the world (with Greece having the highest number of COVID deaths per capita).[24] Total mortality rates in the United States during the COVID epidemic have been about 20 percent above what we would have expected, with approximately one-third of the increase in all-cause US deaths during the pandemic attributable to increases in non-COVID-19 deaths.[25]

As discussed in Chapter 1, SARS-CoV-2 is not eradicable, and so most infectious diseases experts always expected it to become endemic (continually circulating but with rates of severe disease comparable to other respiratory pathogens), thereby leading to an ongoing need for vaccination and therapeutics. But the idea that COVID-19 could be eradicated led to excessive mitigation attempts (as in China, with draconian lockdowns) that had other impacts on public health[26] and on trust in governments (mass protests against COVID restrictions in China erupted in late 2022, leading to re-opening in December 2022).[27]

Vaccines are safe and the most important strategy for preventing severe disease. The biggest contributor to the high mortality from COVID-19 in the United States is the relatively low rate of vaccine uptake (77 percent of people twelve years and older were fully vaccinated by December 2022), especially during the delta surge; this rate compares unfavorably to the rates in European countries and many Latin American countries, where a greater percentage of people had been fully vaccinated.[28] Indeed, the most important predictor of life expectancy loss in a large analysis performed in late 2022 across most European countries, the United States, and Chile seems to be lower vaccination uptake, especially in individuals over sixty years old.[29] And in the United States, excess mortality from COVID-19 seemed to be driven by the states with the lowest vaccination rates.[30]

Another reason for high death rates early on in the United States may have been the failure to protect nursing home residents at that time, given that this infection is most severe for older individuals.[31] An additional early contributor was the failure to protect racial and ethnic minorities from COVID-19, with Black, Latino, and Native American individuals accounting for a disproportionately high number of infections and deaths from early 2020 through June 2022; due to an increase in vaccination rates in minority communities thereafter, COVID deaths among white Americans surpassed those in other groups by mid-2022.[32] The factors that explain the racial/ethnic disparities in deaths early on in the pandemic in the United States include a higher prevalence of comorbid conditions (that is, when a person has other diseases like heart or lung problems), distrust of the medical system (leading to vaccine hesitancy), and socioeconomic determinants that negatively affect health (such as poverty, lack of education, poor housing, the need to rely on public transportation, types of employment that may not support good health, and inadequate access to healthcare).[33] However, community-based messaging and persistent work led to higher vaccination rates among racial/ethnic minorities over time.[34]

Finally, the United States has a fractured healthcare system, with no universal healthcare, underresourced public health services, and especially an inadequate safety net—for example, universal sick leave during COVID-19 was provided by many other countries, but the United States struggled to institute paid sick leave during the pandemic.[35] The fault lines within the US healthcare system were poignantly revealed during the pandemic.[36]

TRANSMISSION

SARS-CoV-2 is primarily transmitted directly from person to person through respiratory particles, both larger droplets and, under certain circumstances, smaller aerosol particles. Transmission principally occurs when respiratory particles containing the virus are released when an infected person coughs, sneezes, or talks in close contact with an uninfected person. SARS-CoV-2 can also be transmitted when airborne in enclosed, poorly ventilated spaces.[37] Moreover, COVID-19 is usually not transmitted through contact with contaminated surfaces.[38] The virus is shed in stool, but fecal-to-oral transmission is not the route of spread for this virus (although sewage surveillance can now serve as a way to track COVID prevalence).[39]

We have learned that longer contact (say, a conversation that lasts more than thirty minutes) and closer contact (such as sharing a bedroom or vehicle) markedly increase transmission. Transmission from infected people who have no symptoms is thought to account for about 19 percent of all transmissions, meaning that transmission from individuals showing symptoms is much more common.[40] Transmission outdoors is incredibly uncommon; a study in Wuhan that involved careful contact tracing discovered that just one of 7,324 infection events investigated was linked to outdoor transmission.[41] Indeed, ventilation has emerged as one of the most important non-pharmaceutical ways to mitigate the spread of COVID-19.[42] Finally, rates of human infection are somewhat lower in parts of the globe that are warmer and sunnier.[43]

It is also possible for humans to transmit SARS-CoV-2 to other mammals. As discussed in Chapter 1, infection has been documented in twenty-nine species of animals to date, including dogs, cats, gorillas, farmed mink, ferrets, hamsters, rabbits, otters, mice, lions, tigers, deer, and others. However, the transmission risk these infected animals pose to humans is still being examined.

After exposure, the incubation period for COVID-19 ranges from two to fourteen days, with onset of symptoms occurring by day twelve in about 98 percent of cases and a relatively constant median of five days among persons without prior immunity or vaccination.[44] Shedding of viable virus (virus that can infect someone else) appears to begin two to three days before the onset of symptoms. It is greatest in the first week of infection, uncommon more than five days after the onset of symptoms, and very unusual by ten days after the onset of symptoms.[45] Vaccination or past infection reduces the length of time someone can infect others after a subsequent breakthrough infection.[46] Since the vast majority of COVID-19 transmissions occur within the first five days, the CDC determined in January 2022 that five days is adequate for a period of isolation following infection (without the need for a negative test).[47] Now that we are in the phase of endemic management, most countries no longer recommend a certain isolation period for COVID-19 but just recommend staying home when sick (a strategy that will minimize the risk of all respiratory pathogen transmission, including colds and flu).[48]

As SARS-CoV-2 has evolved, variants have arisen. Most changes in the virus have little to no impact, but some mutations can change transmissibility, virulence (the severity of disease), the efficacy of therapeutics such as monoclonal antibodies, or the effectiveness of social mitigation measures. If a variant demonstrates increased transmissibility, increased virulence, or an ability to evade the immune system, it is classified as a "variant of concern." The alpha (B.1.1.7), beta (B.1.351), gamma (P.1), delta (B.1.617.2), and omicron (B.1.1.529, with subvariants BA.1, BA.2, BA.2.12.1, BA.3, BA.4, BA.5, BA.2.75, BF.7, BQ.1, BQ1.1, XBB, XBB.1.5, and BA.2.75.2) variants have been designated as variants of concern. For example, the delta variant was more transmissible than the alpha variant but equally virulent.[49] The omicron variant is more transmissible than delta but less virulent.[50] Many of the vaccines initially developed to combat SARS-CoV-2 focused on what's called the spike protein—the feature of the virus that allows it to enter our cells and cause infection. Antibodies generated by the spike-protein-encoding COVID-19 vaccines do not work as well against omicron as they do against other variants; however, T cell immunity generated by vaccines remains effective against all variants to date.[51] (Chapter 3 will get into some of the details of immunology and why omicron drove COVID-19 into endemicity.[52])

SYMPTOMS OF COVID-19
AND WHAT CAUSED THE DISEASE

Prior to the availability of vaccines, patients with SARS-CoV-2 infection had a wide range of clinical symptoms, from as many as

40 percent having no symptoms at all at the start of the pandemic but still testing positive (asymptomatic infection) to a smaller percentage who developed critical illness with respiratory failure. The proportion of asymptomatic infections has increased since the advent of vaccines and with increasing immunity in the population.[53] The only reason people were tested when they did not have any symptoms (which is not usual practice for a respiratory pathogen) is that the spread from asymptomatic individuals early in the pandemic was thought to be very high.[54] However, an important "living" (constantly updated) review shows us that transmission from those without symptoms is approximately two-thirds lower than those with symptoms.[55] This likely puts SARS-CoV-2 on par with other respiratory pathogens (such as influenza), about which we have less extensive data.[56] As with most other viruses, the peak transmission potential of SARS-CoV-2 is likely to be at the onset of symptoms. The fact that the rate of COVID-19 transmission attributable to asymptomatic spread was lower than initially thought—in combination with increasing population immunity— led the United Kingdom to institute updated policies, such as cessation of universal masking in healthcare settings in June 2022 and discontinuation of asymptomatic testing in healthcare settings and nursing homes in August 2022.[57] These policies were also adopted in the United States by the CDC in September 2022, although the CDC tied recommendations about masking in healthcare settings to community transmission rates and restrictions were maintained along political lines.[58]

It's important to note that our testing platforms for SARS-CoV-2 were flawed in that they never measured live virus or the true ability to transmit virus. Polymerase chain reaction (PCR) tests can detect small amounts of dead virus and so can remain positive for up to a hundred days after infection. Antigen tests (rapid tests that use technology similar to that found in over-the-counter pregnancy tests) also do not detect live viruses and can continue to give positive results longer than the person is infectious.[59] Finally, in times when circulating infections are low, the false-positive rate of the antigen tests can be high (with as many as 50 percent of first tests producing false positives), requiring that the tests be repeated for accuracy.[60]

Fever, cough, and loss of taste and smell are the most common symptoms of the COVID-19 variants that emerged before omicron.[61] Other common symptoms include fatigue, muscle aches, sore throat, headache, dry cough, nasal congestion, and shortness of breath. Patients can also progress to very severe COVID-19 pneumonia, respiratory failure, and death, depending on risk factors. With omicron variants, lower respiratory tract symptoms have become less common and gastrointestinal symptoms somewhat more common.[62]

The most striking aspect of COVID-19 is the extent to which severity of disease is associated with increasing age (see the table on page 46), with patients over age sixty-five having the highest risk. As noted earlier, this age distribution is unusual, in that measles, mumps, rubella, diphtheria, pertussis, influenza, respiratory syncytial virus (RSV), and many other pathogens affect young children disproportionately more than older individuals. Although most countries did acknowledge that the risk to children of this particular pandemic was low, the politicization of the pandemic in some regions in the United States led, as we've seen, to unusually prolonged

Figure 1   Risk for COVID-19 Death by Age Group

Age	Death Rate Compared to 18–29-Year-Olds
0–4 years old	Less than the rate
5–17 years old	Less than the rate
18–29 years old	Reference group
30–39 years old	4 times greater rate
40–49 years old	10 times greater rate
50–64 years old	25 times greater rate
65–74 years old	65 times greater rate
75–84 years old	140 times greater rate
85+ years old	330 times greater rate

Source: CDC, "Risk for COVID-19 Infection, Hospitalization, and Death by Age Group," https://www.cdc.gov/coronavirus/2019-ncov/covid-data/investigations -discovery/hospitalization-death-by-age.html, last updated June 2, 2022.

school closures and disruptions for children during COVID-19. The sparing of young children by COVID-19 for severe disease seems to be related to differences in the innate immune response between children and adults, which protects most children from the worst manifestations of the disease.[63]

Important comorbid conditions, which predispose individuals to severe complications (including death) from COVID-19, include diabetes, obesity, cardiovascular disease, kidney disease, chronic lung disease, and sickle cell disease. Most of these are more common in older people. Patients who are transplant recipients, have cancer or uncontrolled HIV infection, or are receiving immuno-suppressive therapy have an increased risk of severe COVID-19. In addition, pregnant women are at increased risk for progression of infection and adverse outcomes. Being unvaccinated without prior immunity is also a significant risk factor for severe illness. At-risk groups need booster vaccinations, should be monitored closely, and should be prioritized for early treatment when available. However, overall, the severity of COVID infections has now decreased markedly with the advent of vaccinations and treatments (including remdesivir, anti-inflammatories, monoclonal antibodies, and oral antivirals such as Paxlovid and molnupiravir), along with rising immunity in the population.[64] An important article in the December 2022 isssue of *Clinical Infectious Diseases* from South Africa showed decreasing cases, hospitalizations, and deaths in the context of the less virulent omicron variant and increasing immunity despite the emergence of subvariants.[65]

PROGNOSIS

In the initial COVID-19 surge caused by the very first COVID-19 strain (Wuhan) in the pre-vaccine era, the infection fatality rate was under 1 percent for persons under age sixty-five but increased to 15 percent for those age eighty-five and older.[66] The severity of the infection has evolved as variants have appeared and as vaccinations have become available for older people. The risk of hospitalization and mortality also have been lower with recent omicron variants than with earlier variants due to inherently lower virulence.[67]

"Primary infection" refers to an infection in someone who is unvaccinated or nonimmune. "Reinfection" refers to getting a second infection after having recovered from a first infection. And "breakthrough infection" refers to an infection occurring in someone who has been vaccinated. Compared to primary infections, reinfections and breakthrough infections rarely lead to hospitalization or death. For instance, in a large CDC analysis conducted from

December 2020 to October 2021 among over 1.2 million adults who had completed the primary vaccination series, the overall rate of severe COVID-19 breakthroughs was 0.015 percent, and the rate of COVID-19 death after a vaccine breakthrough was 0.0033 percent.[68] Risk factors for severe outcomes in this analysis included being sixty-five or older, being immunosuppressed, and having comorbid conditions (of the very small proportion of vaccinated patients who died of COVID-19, 78 percent had at least *four* underlying conditions). A large observational study from Israel showed that those over age sixty-five who were vaccinated were still susceptible to severe breakthrough infections, requiring an antiviral to treat.[69] The largest analysis of who remained at risk for severe disease after two-dose vaccination was published in October 2022 in *The Lancet*; this large UK analysis examining 30 million people who had severe breakthrough infections showed that being eighty years or older, having chronic kidney disease, being on immunosuppressants, and having five or more other medical conditions were risk factors for severe COVID-19 disease.[70] These kinds of population-level studies allow the public health community to target those at risk of severe breakthroughs (including older patients and those on immunosuppressants) for booster vaccination and treatment (for example, oral antivirals like Paxlovid).[71]

Most patients who have had COVID-19 recover completely, but some patients experience prolonged symptoms or develop long-term effects.[72] The WHO defines this condition—PASC, also commonly called long COVID—as symptoms that persist for at least two months after resolution of probable or confirmed acute SARS-CoV-2 infection (i.e., usually three months after the onset of

COVID-19) and that cannot be explained by an alternative diagnosis. The CDC, by comparison, defines PASC as new, returning, or ongoing health problems four or more weeks after first being infected with SARS-CoV-2. PASC is rare in children and seems to be much more common in patients who initially experienced severe COVID-19.[73] A longitudinal National Institutes of Health (NIH) study of those with PASC did not find major differences in inflammatory markers or autoantibodies between those recovering from COVID-19 and those without COVID-19, and it also found that symptoms were more common in women than men.[74] Residual symptoms for some time after severe respiratory illness have been reported with many other viral pathogens and were reported to be lower with COVID-19 than with severe respiratory illness from other pathogens during the pandemic.[75] Data suggests that long COVID symptoms are no more common in vaccinated people who've had a breakthrough infection than they are in uninfected control patients, thereby indicating that vaccination is highly protective against PASC.[76] Because, as we've seen, long COVID symptoms are most clearly associated with an initial diagnosis of severe COVID, growing population immunity over time (which decreases the likelihood of severe disease) has decreased the incidence of the condition significantly.[77] Studies are ongoing to help us determine the best way to treat people who develop PASC, although antihistamines, fluvoxamine, and the antiviral Paxlovid have all had early success.

The rate of severe disease in children from COVID-19, as discussed previously, is markedly lower than that among adults. The United Kingdom provided the best data on pediatric disease, as the CDC unfortunately was plagued by data coding errors, problems with data transparency, and programming errors during COVID-19.[78] The UK National Health Service—which is a universal healthcare system with centralized reporting—allowed researchers there to collect more accurate data than was possible in the United States. In the United Kingdom, among about 12 million children and adolescents younger than twenty, there were eighty-one recorded COVID-19 deaths over the first two years of the pandemic, providing an infection fatality rate of 0.70/100,000 infections (that is, 0.0007 percent).[79] Moreover, of these eighty-one deaths, sixty-one (or 75.3 percent) occurred among children with underlying conditions, especially severe neurodisability and immunocompromising conditions. This rate contrasts sharply with the 1 percent mortality rate among adults over fifty prior to vaccines in the United Kingdom.[80]

PREVENTION OF SARS-COV-2 PRIOR TO VACCINES

Prior to the availability of vaccines and monoclonal antibodies, the strategies that were recommended to minimize transmission were physical distancing, face masks, ventilation, avoidance of indoor gatherings, testing, and contact tracing.[81] (Ventilation, which is such an important mitigation procedure for COVID-19, is something we will need to emphasize in the future for all pathogens that affect the respiratory system.)[82]

After vaccines became available in high-income countries and after the milder omicron variant emerged, almost all countries eventually abandoned more drastic ways to decrease transmission, such as lockdowns, since hospital capacity was no longer strained the way it had been early in the pandemic. Moreover, lockdowns had many detrimental effects globally, including on adults' mental health, poverty, hunger, control of other communicable (such as tuberculosis, malaria, and HIV) and non-communicable diseases (such as cardiovascular health and cancer), children's mental and physical health and educational attainment, and economies.[83] China maintained the longest duration of COVID-zero policies, with rolling lockdowns and mass testing. After a tragic fire killed 10 people who couldn't leave their building due to lockdowns in November 2022, mass protests against COVID-zero erupted on the streets of Chinese cities and the country changed its approach in December.[84]

FACE MASKS AS MITIGATION
STRATEGIES FOR THE PUBLIC

Since universal face masking was the most controversial measure introduced during the COVID-19 pandemic, it is important to spend some time covering the data behind this almost universally applied intervention. In the spring of 2020, various restrictions and interventions, including mask mandates, made sense—even sometimes in the absence of rigorous science supporting them.[85] That was understandable at the time; indeed, I wrote one of the first papers calling for universal face masks to help prevent transmission of COVID-19.[86]

Our group had a hypothesis that face masks reduced the number of viral particles reaching a person's system and that this would lead to less severe disease early on in the pandemic. Later studies showed that this hypothesis was on the right track.[87] For instance, a Hong Kong study showed that masks didn't decrease transmission but increased the percentage of infections that were asymptomatic, perhaps because people who masked were exposed to less virus.[88] A study in nonhuman primates showed that the higher the dose of SARS-CoV-2, the greater the severity of disease.[89] And NIH researchers provided evidence that the increased humidity behind cloth masks may lessen the severity of disease.[90] However, the best way to reduce severity of disease is to get vaccinated, so this benefit became negligible as vaccines became available.

The next question was whether masks reduced transmission and saved lives. In the Hong Kong study mentioned above, the data does not show that masks made an appreciable difference in transmission at the population level. A large-cluster randomized controlled trial (where villages were randomized to masking or not) conducted in six hundred villages in Bangladesh showed a small but statistically significant benefit: among people who consistently used masks, 7.6 percent reported symptomatic infections, compared to 8.6 percent in the control group.[91] But this study included both self-reported "COVID-like symptoms" and positive COVID serology tests, and so the absolute reduction was a bit smaller. Moreover, a re-analysis of the raw data from the study did not show even this small benefit.[92] Other studies that used a randomized controlled format have also not shown the effectiveness of face masks in reducing the spread of respiratory pathogens.[93] Observational studies have not convincingly shown that mask mandates improved outcomes in the US states that had them compared to states that did not, in terms of either total cases or hospitalizations. Most well-done studies do not show an association between mask mandates and the containment of spread or a reduction in hospitalizations.[94] This may seem counterintuitive, but it could be because mask-wearing practices and types of masks vary so that individual-level benefits of masks can occur without population-level mask mandates being effective.

I think it was justified to try universal face masking prior to the widespread availability of vaccines for a new pathogen, but mandating face masks after vaccinations were widely available did not have solid evidence behind it and intensified polarization. During the delta surge, California counties with mask mandates fared no better than those without mask mandates in terms of cases and hospitalizations if vaccination rates were similar.[95] In states with and without mask mandates during the omicron surge, cases predictably rose and dropped at the same rate, likely because getting infected increases antibody levels in your nasal passages and reduces your chance of onward transmission, whether masked or not.[96]

Since the omicron variant was so transmissible, efforts at universal contact tracing were dropped by the CDC in March 2022.[97] In addition, studies showed that universal testing and mask mandates did not contain the spread of omicron on a college campus (although vaccines continued to work well).[98] Basically, the idea that masks protect others has not been borne out by studies, and mask mandates themselves don't seem to work to curb the spread of the disease.[99] As discussed previously, this is likely because people wear different kinds of masks and wear them in different ways (e.g., below the nose). Indeed, studies using mannequins show that well-fitted good-quality masks (like N95, KN95, FFP2, and KF94 masks) do seem to work in indoor spaces to block respiratory pathogens from reaching the individual and can be recommended to vulnerable individuals moving forward in indoor crowded places.[100]

Finally, keeping mask mandates in place after vaccines were available in the United States didn't make sense, since all of the restrictions imposed earlier in the pandemic (masking, testing, distancing, contact tracing, et cetera) were aimed at lowering transmission and the subsequent burden on hospitals until we could get to a vaccine, the most effective way to prevent severe disease. In countries such as Denmark and the United Kingdom, which dropped restrictions after vaccines became available, unlike in Democratic-led areas in the United States, the public seemed to have higher levels of trust in public health authorities.[101]

FACE MASKS FOR CHILDREN

If public masking was polarizing in the United States, the issue of prolonged masking of young children in schools was even more contentious. The CDC drew on four studies to say that "masks work" in schools, but the studies were flawed, especially where they didn't take into account vaccination rates in the community after vaccines became available.[102] A well-done study performed in Catalonia, Spain, showed that face masks in children did not work at all to reduce transmission; the chance of COVID infection was dependent on the age of the child and not on whether the school used masks.[103]

In terms of masks for the very young, the CDC was an outlier in recommending that children less than five years old mask. The WHO has in fact recommended against masking children under age six, and Scandinavia has, during the entire pandemic, never required masks for children under age twelve (and the rates of severe disease in children and teachers in Scandinavian countries were similar to those in other countries).[104] When faces are partially hidden, children's natural learning is compromised.[105] This is especially true for the youngest children, for those with special needs, and for those learning English as a second language.[106] We know from studies of children who are blind that language and emotional development may be hindered by lack of visual cues.[107] It will likely take years to determine the impacts of masking on children's development, but some studies have already found negative effects on early childhood development and language when the adults interacting with the children are wearing masks.[108] Other studies have shown that facial occlusion (in this case, due to mask wearing by teachers) negatively impacts the ability of children to read emotions accurately.[109] And the United Kingdom released data on April 4, 2022, showing that COVID restrictions have set back early childhood personal, social, and emotional development.[110] A study published in October 2022 found that Irish infants born from March to May 2020 had a harder time communicating (e.g., waving goodbye, saying their first word, pointing to objects) at one year of age than those born before the pandemic.[111]

Therefore, normalizing children's lives became a major strategic initiative after the World Health Organization, the European CDC, and US public health officials called the emergency phase of the pandemic over, noting that the endemic phase had begun.[112] The United Kingdom and most European countries had already dropped all restrictions on children in the early spring of 2022, but the CDC—despite revised school guidance in August 2022 that paved the way for fewer school disruptions than in 2021—continued restrictions such as intermittent masking in schools based on exposure and asymptomatic surveillance testing in areas with high community transmission.[113] However, by the fall of 2022, after a prominent infectious diseases journal published a reanalysis of CDC data showing that masking schoolchildren actually offered no benefit, an accompanying editorial by a prominent scientist in COVID-19 mitigation said that masking children for COVID-19 should be permanently discontinued.[114] Other UK-based pediatricians—concerned about the potential for harms of masks in developing children—wrote papers along the same lines that fall.[115]

MOVING ON FROM THE EMERGENCY
PHASE OF THE PANDEMIC

In March 2022, the WHO laid out a plan to begin moving on from the emergency phase of the response to COVID-19.[116] The next month, the European CDC called for endemic management of COVID-19.[117] In the United States, the CDC did not change its guidelines to reflect endemic management, given high rates of population immunity, until August 2022.[118] And in September, the WHO said the end of the pandemic "was in sight."[119] Yet it was unclear what these proclamations meant. Because SARS-CoV-2 is a non-eradicable virus, COVID-19 will never be over, but it was clear that, given the impact of the COVID-19 response on other public health goals, we had to move on from the emergency phase of management. What we needed was a plan to manage an endemic virus.[120]

CHAPTER 3

How Do We Manage COVID-19 Now?

As we've discussed, SARS-CoV-2, unlike smallpox, is not eradicable.[1] For one thing, as noted, at least twenty-nine species of animals can harbor the virus, and any virus with such extensive animal reservoirs cannot be eradicated worldwide.[2] Not that some authorities haven't tried eliminating these animal reservoirs; some violent episodes with animals during the COVID-19 pandemic included the slaughter of 17 million mink in Denmark in November 2020 after the mink were found to carry coronavirus; the culling of pet hamsters in Hong Kong in November 2021; and the killing of pet dogs and cats in China as late as spring 2022.[3] I remember hearing in April 2020 that big cats in a New York zoo were found to have COVID-19.[4] I knew then that we will never eradicate the virus and that we needed to get to a phase of control, where population immunity, vaccines, and therapeutics controlled severe disease.

ENDEMIC MANAGEMENT FOR COVID-19 CAME IN FITS AND STARTS IN 2022

The ancestral strain of the virus was first identified in January 2020.[5] There was a variant, D614G, that became the dominant strain in the summer of 2020 but never got its own Greek letter designation.[6] The alpha variant became a worldwide variant in late 2020 and early

2021, but the beta (first detected in South Africa) and gamma (first identified in Brazil) variants stayed relatively confined to certain geographical areas, since they were less transmissible than previous strains.[7] The delta variant, first identified in India in March 2021, was extremely transmissible and just as deadly as earlier variants; it led to terrible death and suffering in India, which had only a 4 percent vaccination rate at the time.[8] But the omicron variant—which was first identified by South African scientists in mid-November 2021—was different.[9] Omicron could not infect lung cells as effectively as previous variants, making it a more "feeble" variant.[10]

In the United States, COVID-19 vaccination was still extremely protective against hospitalization from the omicron variant, as it had been against the delta variant.[11] However, there are estimates that by March 2022 over 60 percent of the world's population had been exposed to omicron and its subvariants, leading to a great deal of immunity in the population.[12] The CDC reported on April 26, 2022 (drawing on data through February 2022), that 60 percent of the adult population of the United States and 75 percent of children up to age eighteen had been exposed to COVID-19, as measured by the nucleocapsid antibody, which is not generated by the vaccines but only by natural infection.[13] Just a few months later, in August, the seroprevalence (rate of natural infection) among children in the United States rose to 86 percent.[14] This population immunity, combined with worldwide dissemination of the vaccines since January 2021, led to the low number of deaths from COVID-19 seen in the spring of 2022. All this was what led up to the April 2022 statements by the WHO, the European CDC, and US public health officials that the emergency phase of the pandemic was ending.[15]

However, although Europe stayed true to its promise to enter the endemic phase of management for COVID-19 in the spring of 2022 (acknowledging that other aspects of public health had been neglected), it took several more months, until August, for the CDC to change its guidance to acknowledge the high levels of both vaccine-induced and natural immunity.[16]

None of this meant that the controversy over COVID-19 in the United States was over. Some US public health experts came out against the CDC's new guidance in August 2022; there was a storm when a prominent CNN and *Washington Post* commentator who was a physician endorsed the guidelines; and some blue states, like California, ignored the CDC guidance in favor of continuing asymptomatic testing and school masking. All this spoke to our polarization along party lines around COVID-19.[17] The *New England Journal of Medicine* published a piece that month pleading with public health practitioners to consider nuance and trade-offs in their recommendations, arguing that "complex decisions" like mask mandates "should be widely and publicly debated by public health institutions . . . and it would behoove public health practitioners to stop suggesting in social media posts that nuanced questions have universally correct answers."[18]

I couldn't have agreed more with the *New England Journal of Medicine* piece urging nuance and acknowledging trade-offs in our COVID pandemic response, especially given the evolving science. Nearly a year earlier, in November 2021, several public health practitioners and I wrote a piece about ten evidence-based policies for COVID-19 management (these form the basis of the pandemic preparedness I discuss in the final chapter).[19] In March 2022, the director of UCSF's emergency room response to COVID-19 and I wrote a piece about a "rational road map" to managing COVID-19 in the future.[20] Specifically, we suggested the following:

1. Discontinuing mass asymptomatic testing and quarantines, especially in schools, but maintaining wastewater surveillance.

2. Continuing the five-day isolation period for people after they test positive for COVID-19 and asking people to stay home when sick.

3. Investing in a test-and-treat program, so that we can more effectively use antivirals in those who are unvaccinated and at risk of severe infection or in those who are vaccinated and at risk of a severe breakthrough.

4. Acknowledging natural infection in our vaccination strategies as well as discontinuing the divisive strategies of vaccine mandates and vaccine "passports," since—with the newer variants—transmission can occur even from vaccinated people.

5. Extending the interval between vaccination doses for the primary series to at least eight weeks.

6. Clarifying our vaccine booster strategy to focus on preventing severe disease, not trying to chase the impossible goal of preventing every infection.

7. Expanding our vaccine arsenal in the United States to include Novavax (a more traditional protein-based vaccine) and Covaxin (an inactivated whole-virus vaccine) (discussed later in this chapter).

8. Discussing how vaccines can help prevent the symptoms of PASC (long COVID) by reducing severe disease, which is most closely associated with post-COVID symptoms.

9. Continuing to upgrade and improve ventilation systems for indoor spaces.

10. Retiring mask mandates for good in favor of recommendations of fit and filtered masks for vulnerable individuals.

This piece on endemic management was the culmination of others I'd written (most often with other public health experts) about why overcaution regarding COVID-19, especially with the availability of vaccines for teachers, carried its own risk for schoolchildren. Mass asymptomatic testing in schools was leading to too much learning loss; quarantines kept children out of school too long; and school closures were having negative effects on teen mental health. I'd been pointing out that we would never be able to eradicate COVID-19, so we would have to gain immunity (preferably through vaccination) to usher in the endemic phase. Once we had vaccines, I emphasized that hospitalizations were the most important metric to keep track of and urged that restrictions should be reimagined after vaccines became available.[21]

I believe it is partially because of the hope that COVID-19 could be eradicated that the United States remained polarized around COVID-19 throughout 2022, especially with China still pursuing a COVID-zero strategy.[22] However, most other countries were working on reducing severe disease (not infections) to as low as possible, with the United Kingdom reporting in March 2022 that its COVID-19 mortality rate was lower than the mortality rate from influenza in a typical year, despite the discontinuation of most restrictions in the UK in July 2021.[23]

Another factor that affected the United States but not most other countries when the omicron variant hit our shores was the CDC's problems with data collection, including issues with data transparency.[24] Many US leaders failed to recognize the power of immunity, and this was in large part due to a data problem regarding the misclassification of hospitalizations.[25] Even as immunity rose in the population and with a less virulent variant, we were continuing to miscategorize a large number of hospitalizations as being "from COVID" rather than "with COVID" (just swabbing positive for COVID but being hospitalized for something else).[26] As early as February 2022, the Biden administration indicated they wanted to make sure hospitalizations were classified accurately.[27] Despite this, the misclassification trend continued further into 2022, making it appear that COVID mortality was still much higher than influenza mortality, even though that was no longer the case.[28] Classification of deaths as occuring from COVID-19 when they did not can make immunity and the vaccines look less powerful (which is why mass asymptomatic testing of hospitalized patients ended in the United Kingdom and other countries in August 2022). The mistaken impression that immunity and the vaccines were not as effective as they really were, due to this practice of asymptomatic screening in the United States, may have contributed to the polarization in this country. Only in late December 2022 did the Society for Healthcare Epidemiology of America finally recommended that hospitals stop screening every asymptomatic inpatient admission for SARS-CoV-2, a practice change that should allow hospitalizations to be properly classified.[29]

HOW DOES CELLULAR IMMUNITY WORK?

Let's take a brief detour to look more closely at why, exactly, immunity and vaccines are so effective.

Antibodies are one arm of the immune system. They're generated by infection or vaccines. Over time, however, antibodies wane. Luckily, vaccines or infections also generate something called cellular immunity (B and T cells), which are much longer-lasting and protect against severe disease in a more enduring fashion.[30]

Memory B cells—whether generated by the vaccines or as a result of a prior infection—have been shown to recognize the virus, including its variants.[31] Think of memory B cells as a recipe that can make more antibodies if they see the virus in the future. If memory B cells encounter a variant, they are able to make antibodies adapted to that particular variant.[32] Although we do not yet know for sure how long these memory B cells will be able to recognize COVID-19, we do know that elderly survivors of the 1918 influenza pandemic (ages 91 to 101) were able to produce antibodies from memory B cells when their blood was exposed to the same strain nine decades later.[33]

The vaccines or natural infection also trigger the production of T cells.[34] While B cells serve as memory banks to produce antibodies when needed, T cells both help B cells make antibodies and help recruit other immune-system cells to attack the pathogen directly. Memory T cells generated by COVID-19 infection may last a lifetime, according to a study that examined people who had had infections of varying degrees of severity.[35] Memory T cells generated in individuals who survived a different coronavirus infection in 2003 (SARS, covered in Chapter 2) have been shown to last at least seventeen years.[36]

During the omicron subvariant surges in spring 2022, we did see a greater chance of reinfection compared with previous variants—but no increase in severe disease across the general population.[37] This defanging of the virus was even more evident upon closer analysis of hospitalization data. In states like Massachusetts that track hospitalization in detail, there was a clear trend showing that the majority of hospital patients who tested positive for COVID were being hospitalized for reasons other than COVID— the discovery of their infection was merely incidental.[38] A study from Southern California showed similarly that two-thirds of hospital patients testing positive for COVID had been hospitalized for another reason.[39] By November 2022, daily confirmed deaths from COVID-19 globally were 90 percent down from the beginning of the year.[40]

HOW DO WE KEEP COVID-19
IN THE ENDEMIC PHASE?

Now that COVID-19 is in the endemic phase, rather than the emergency pandemic phase, how do we keep the disease at manageable levels?

VACCINES

The initial vaccines were developed to combat the specific variants of the disease seen early on in the pandemic, and we have been lucky that these vaccines continue to be protective against severe disease and hospitalization even now that we have omicron and its subvariants, which are better able to evade the antibodies of the immune system.[41] However, the omicron lineage led to a lot of mild infections across the planet in the spring of 2022, and so vaccine developers altered their targets. By the fall of 2022, we had omicron-specific mRNA vaccines available in the United States.[42]

The reason that prior infection or vaccination protects against severe disease is cellular immunity.[43] When you get a vaccine, your body produces antibodies that neutralize the virus; in the medical field, this is called humoral immunity, and it's the first line of defense against infection. When we get updated vaccines, we produce new antibodies that are targeted to the latest versions of the virus. But, as we've seen, antibodies wane over time, and the ones generated by the vaccines don't work as well against new variants. This is where T cells and memory B cells come in.[44] A study of the Pfizer vaccine, which was developed before omicron became prevalent, showed that Pfizer vaccine–induced T cells also respond to the omicron variant, continuing to bind and help kill it even though it is in many respects different from the earlier variants.[45] Protection from severe disease remains strong in vaccinated people because a breakthrough infection spurs the body to respond with both humoral and T cell immunity.[46] And even though antibodies decline after either a booster or a breakthrough infection, memory B cells exhibit broad-spectrum adaptation to the variant to which they are exposed and quickly generate antibodies specific to the variant they're encountering.[47]

Older individuals, whose immune systems tend to be less robust, and those with immunocompromising conditions need boosting. South Korea has very high rates of boosting among the country's elderly, and during the BA1 surge this provided important protection against hospitalizations and deaths.[48] The world needs to aggressively double down on the importance of boosters for the elderly. A large Veterans Affairs study of older patients (median age seventy-one) during the omicron surge in the United States showed that those who had received three doses of vaccine—the two-shot primary series plus one booster—had a lower rate of hospitalization and less need for ICU-level care than those with only the two doses of the primary series.[49]

Second boosters were approved for Americans over the age of fifty in the United States in March 2021. Although the antibodies from the second booster (which was the mRNA vaccine formulated for the old strain) unfortunately waned faster than the antibodies from the first booster, each booster (or exposure) diversifies and broadens T cell responses to the virus, and a booster shot in particular will also expand the potency of B cells.[50] Therefore, boosters are important for those at high risk for severe COVID-19 and will be needed on an ongoing basis for vulnerable individuals. Updated omicron-specific mRNA vaccines became available across Canada, Europe, and the United States in the fall of 2022, and boosters for older people were especially strongly encouraged.[51]

Finally, what's called hybrid immunity (either infection after vaccination or vaccination after infection) provided stronger protection than vaccine or infection alone, as shown in multiple epidemiological studies.[52] When someone who's been vaccinated gets a breakthrough infection, they develop broad neutralizing antibodies against reinfection with other subvariants; antibodies and T cells begin to patrol the nose and mouth, the areas where virus particles enter the body; and the immune system trains up T cells.[53] Multiple epidemiological and immunological studies show that a breakthrough infection in vaccinated people counts as a "booster," and so an additional booster shot of vaccine is not necessary for most of these people. But all older people worldwide, even those who have had a natural infection, should at least get one dose of the vaccine to strengthen their immune response.[54]

By June 2022, the United States had approved vaccines for children down to the age of six months. And, as was just mentioned, in the fall of 2022 an omicron-specific booster was approved (although many scientists argued that boosters should be reserved for older individuals, given the increased risk of severe breakthroughs in this population).[55] But all these are mRNA vaccines, so let's take a quick look at how they work.

The mRNA vaccine technology uses a type of protein that exists in the cells of all living organisms. This protein is a code that tells the body how to produce other types of protein. When creating an mRNA vaccine, scientists use pieces of mRNA that code for part of the SARS-CoV-2 virus's spike protein (and, as we've seen, the spike protein is the tool the virus uses to get inside our cells and cause an infection). After we receive the vaccine, our body translates that genetic material and makes some of the spike protein. The immune system then recognizes that spike protein as an invader and raises an immune response to it. Then the mRNA and the spike protein our body has created both get broken down, leaving behind a powerful immune arsenal of T cells, B cells, and antibodies.[56]

These mRNA vaccines were a new type of vaccine. More traditional vaccines, like those used to protect against influenza, pertussis (whooping cough), diphtheria, and tetanus, are what's called protein subunit vaccines; they use fragments of proteins from the disease-causing virus to trigger the immune system. Because the mRNA vaccines were so different, some people felt hesitant to get them. A good proportion of this hesitancy arose because of misinformation from many sources, including word of mouth, social media platforms, television, and popular entertainment and media organizations.[57] The WHO actually described it best: with too much information—some of it false or misleading—circulating online and in other media during the pandemic, we were suffering from an "infodemic." This can cause confusion, lead people to take risks that threaten their health, and sow mistrust of medical authorities and public health agencies.[58]

Whether because of this misinformation or for some other reason, many Americans chose not to receive the mRNA vaccines when they first became available. In fact, as noted, the United States, with only 77 percent of those twelve and older having been fully vaccinated as of December 2022, has lower rates of COVID-19 vaccination than many Latin American and European countries.[59] And the United States was slower than other countries to expand its vaccine arsenal beyond these mRNA vaccines.[60]

But additional vaccine types have now been marketed or are in development. One of them is Novavax (NVX-CoV2373), the more traditional protein subunit vaccine whose use we began advocating in November 2021. The hope was that this vaccine could overcome some Americans' hesitancy about vaccination.[61] The Novavax vaccine was reviewed by the FDA's Vaccines and Available Biological Products Advisory Committee on June 7, 2022, and was granted emergency use authorization (EUA) status soon thereafter, with authorization for Novavax to be given as a booster in October.[62] The Novavax vaccine has been shown to produce strong T cell and antibody responses.[63] (To get technical: NVX-CoV2373 contains a recombinant SARS-CoV-2 nanoparticle vaccine, constructed from the full-length wild-type SARS-CoV-2 spike protein, including the receptor binding domain, or RBD—the piece of the protein that binds directly to the host cell.[64]) The Novavax vaccine comes co-formulated with a Matrix-M1 adjuvant, which is an ingredient added to the vaccine to generate a stronger immune response.[65] However, by the fall of 2022, population immunity was so high in the United States that not many people opted for the Novavax vaccine.

The Covaxin vaccine may be the next vaccine approved in the United States if all goes well with a current trial. Covaxin is one of three vaccines on the WHO list that are inactivated whole-virus vaccines combined with different adjuvants; the two others are Sinopharm and Sinovac (both made in China). Covaxin was originally developed in India by a company named Bharat Pharmaceuticals but now has a US manufacturer named Ocugen.[66] With an inactivated (killed) whole-virus vaccine, the body sees the entire virus and develops an immune response across multiple parts of it. Of these three whole-virus vaccines, Covaxin seems to be the most capable of creating a strong immune response with just two doses (the WHO recommends a third shot for populations receiving Sinopharm and Sinovac).[67] Covaxin's advantage over the two Chinese-made vaccines is likely due to a more powerful adjuvant used in the compound, an adjuvant developed with funding by the US National Institutes of Health.[68]

In addition to encouraging vaccination among people who might be hesitant to get an mRNA vaccine, there are other reasons to develop new vaccines. As we've seen, the initial mRNA vaccines targeted SARS-CoV-2's spike protein. But since then, new variants of concern have emerged that show many mutations to the spike protein. Given this, boosters that show our immune system the entire virus may be useful in generating a broader immune response against variants. In fact, data has shown that getting a Covaxin booster after receiving other vaccines allows the body to neutralize both the delta and omicron variants, so this gives Covaxin a potential advantage when used as a booster against future variants.[69]

You might be wondering why Covaxin isn't yet available in the United States, at least as of this writing. The vaccine's manufacturer, Ocugen, applied to the FDA for authorization for Covaxin to be given to children ages two to eighteen, but the FDA denied that application on March 4, 2022, since the vaccine has mainly been administered in India and not in US populations, and the FDA wanted to see US data.[70] So Ocugen launched a phase 2/3 trial in the United States among four hundred adults beginning in February 2022 and completed enrollment for the trial in August.[71] If Covaxin is safe and boosts antibodies in this US-based population, the vaccine should be authorized after the trial is completed. (On a personal note: I had received three mRNA vaccine shots by the summer of 2022 but had not contracted COVID-19. Because I was traveling to India for a prolonged period that summer to place my husband's ashes in the Ganges, I took the Covaxin vaccine in India in August 2022 as a booster.)

Finally, to prevent even mild infections, multiple nasal spray vaccines in development might hold the answer. While shots in the arm do a great job protecting us from severe illness by inducing the production of T cells and memory B cells, they often can't mount a fast enough mobilization of immune defenses to our throats and nasal passages when we are initially exposed to the virus. This is problematic in the face of the omicron subvariants, which are more efficient at replicating in the upper airways than previous variants.[72] But spraying our nose with a vaccine could station immune responses in our upper respiratory passages to stop the virus from ever entering our cells in the first place.

THERAPEUTICS

Vaccines have allowed us to significantly bolster our defenses against severe illness and death. With therapeutics such as oral antivirals and monoclonal antibody treatments, we can add another layer of protection and keep high-risk vaccinated and unvaccinated people out of the hospital. But we must ensure that both the public and physicians are aware of these treatment options, and we must make them easy to access.

In initial study data, the oral antiviral Paxlovid (which combines two different drugs, nirmatrelvir and ritonavir) demonstrated nearly 90 percent effectiveness at preventing hospitalization in unvaccinated trial participants.[73] And now we have real-world data out of Israel showing a clear benefit from Paxlovid in those at high risk for severe COVID disease (65 and older with comorbidities), vaccinated or not.[74] Even against the more immune-evasive omicron variant, in those over sixty-five there was an 81 percent reduction in deaths and a 67 percent reduction in hospitalizations. Data from the CDC in May 2022 confirmed that Paxlovid was highly effective in preventing severe disease in those at risk of a severe breakthrough infection, with fewer than 1 percent needing hospitalization or a trip to the emergency department after a five-day course of Paxlovid.[75] And the largest study on the use of Paxlovid in vaccinated patients, published in September 2022, showed that the drug reduced hospitalizations and deaths for those over sixty-five years of age with comorbidities though it showed no benefit for those forty to sixty-four years old.[76]

The oral antiviral molnupiravir has taken a back seat to Paxlovid so far. However, it has fewer interactions with other drugs than Paxlovid does. Molnupiravir demonstrated a 30 percent reduction in hospitalization or death among unvaccinated patients and a greater benefit among those who are immunocompromised.[77] Molnupiravir does not seem to benefit those who are vaccinated, according to a large UK study called PANORAMIC, conducted among mainly people less than sixty-five years of age.[78] As discussed earlier, the newest omicron subvariants did not respond to previous monocolonal antibody treatments, but new monoclonal antibody treatments are in development.[79]

And finally, as of this writing, although monoclonal antibodies were employed for treatment or prophylaxis for severely immunocompromised patients from 2020 to 2022, the new omicron sub-variants rendered them ineffective and more are now in development. I need to first emphasize that the COVID-19 vaccines actually work better among immunocompromised patients than the media ever indicated—one of the biggest failures of media coverage of COVID-19, in my estimation.[80] This is probably because the mRNA vaccines raise such a strong and redundant immune response. A large study showed that a primary vaccine series and booster was very effective for patients on immunosuppressant treatment for rheumatological disorders.[81] During the delta variant, three doses of an mRNA vaccine gave immunocompromised individuals 87 percent protection against hospitalization (compared to 97 percent for the general population); this study also showed that the Moderna vaccine stimulated a stronger immune response than the Pfizer vaccine, probably due to the former vaccine's higher dose. Furthermore, in a large study of those on chemotherapy for solid organ tumors, T cell responses to the vaccines were maintained at a high level, although a boost of antibodies during the treatment is certainly important.[82] Immunocompromised individuals were approved for a fourth COVID-19 shot in the spring of 2021 and will need a booster annually.[83]

But for those immunocompromised patients who have undergone solid organ transplants or who are on B-cell-depleting therapies and thus are unable to mount a significant protective response from vaccination, we have been recommending the long-acting dual-monoclonal antibody Evusheld (tixagevimab co-packaged with cilgavimab) for prophylaxis.[84] Given as pre-exposure prophylaxis, Evusheld can provide protection for upward of six months to immunocompromised patients. Evusheld has been shown to be effective against subvariants BA.4 and BA.5 as well, although not against variant BA4.6 and the other new subvariants. As of this writing, Evusheld is still approved for the severely immunocompromised as a protective agent for COVID-19.[85]

None of these treatments (or any of the others now in development) will be helpful if people can't get access to them, however. So, in the spring of 2022, the White House significantly increased the supply of Paxlovid available at test-to-treat hubs, mainly pharmacies. Test to treat just means that pharmacies will have the ability to both test a patient for COVID-19 and dispense Paxlovid if the patient is at a high risk of progression to severe disease. And we have made tremendous progress in terms of giving physicians the information they need to feel confident about managing interactions between COVID-19 treatments and other drugs in their high-risk patients.

INCREASING TRUST IN PUBLIC HEALTH

Voter backlash to school closures in the United States was thought to have played some role in the November 2020 elections.[86] Moreover, we should all be concerned by the mounting evidence that mistrust of public health officials in the United States impacted people's willingness to get vaccines for COVID-19 and, more recently, for other vaccine-preventable diseases.[87] A US study in June 2022 demonstrated an association between low COVID vaccine uptake and decreased influenza vaccine acceptance compared to prior years.[88] Polio vaccination rates among children in some US counties are now less than 60 percent.[89] And the first case of paralytic polio since

2013 was reported in New York in June 2022, leading the state to declare a health emergency in September.[90] A measles outbreak was reported in Maricopa County, Arizona, in August, and a daycare measles outbreak was reported in Ohio in November.[91] Another consequence of the public's lack of trust in health experts is that some people avoid medical care; this may have a more serious impact on communities of color.[92]

———

The terrible losses from the pandemic should not be minimized. But there have also been immense harms from the mitigation strategies designed to slow the spread of COVID, and it is time to strike the right balance between fighting the virus and returning to normalcy in society.[93] To do so, we need to restore our nation's health experts to a position of trusted authority and bring the United States toward one goal: collective health and well-being.

CHAPTER 4

Resources Before Restrictions and the Duty of Public Health

B efore we address the impact of school closures in Chapter 5, the duty of the public health community to ensure global access to therapeutics and vaccines in Chapter 6, and a post-pandemic playbook in Chapter 7, it is worth revisiting the basic principles of public health. In the United States, during and even after the emergency phase of COVID-19, when we think of public health, we may think of dictums such as wearing a mask. But public health is far more than just simple fixes. Rather, it involves the hard work of building an equitable healthcare system. This means ensuring that all populations (not just the wealthy) have high-quality care. The lessons of COVID-19 can help lead us toward that goal.[1]

Together with public health experts from UCSF and Johns Hopkins University, in July 2021 I wrote a piece for the *British Medical Journal* blog on the duty of public health.[2] We introduced the piece this way:

Public health has traditionally operated on core principles including equity, social justice, and participation. Equity is critical since the impact of respiratory pathogens ha[s] historically been defined by socioeconomic disparities. These disparities, therefore, could have been anticipated as drivers of COVID-19. Social justice suggests the need to try and achieve balance of the benefit and potential harms of an intervention to a community. And finally, participation focuses on engaging beneficiaries in the design and implementation of public health programmes.

In the rest of this chapter, I'll go through the points we addressed in that piece.

RESOURCES BEFORE RESTRICTIONS

The first principle we discussed in our essay was *resources before restrictions*. I've mentioned this before; it involves giving people the information and tools they need to stay safe, rather than imposing stringent blanket restrictions that have numerous negative consequences. In the earliest stages of the pandemic, when we were facing a highly transmissible respiratory virus we knew very little about, it was tempting to try to lock down the planet, the argument being that keeping people away from each other was the best way to minimize transmission. And certainly these early lockdowns allowed us to figure out how the pathogen spread and to develop mitigation procedures such as testing, contact tracing, masking, ventilation, and distancing. So, lockdowns seemed like a reasonable way to reduce the burden on hospitals that were having to cope with a novel virus in a population that had no immunity to it. Lockdowns were meant to last only for a short period, until the mechanisms of transmission were figured out, but were extended in many places.

Extended lockdowns hurt the poor the most.[3] This fact was clear early on during the COVID-19 pandemic and from earlier pandemics. In the 1918 influenza pandemic, the inability to work from home, lack of pay when absent from work, and self-employment were all associated with an inability to comply with public health mitigation recommendations.[4] In India in March 2020, Prime Minister Narendra Modi abruptly ordered a lockdown of 1.38 billion people, leading millions in poverty to struggle for food and thousands of migrant workers to start walking from urban centers to their ancestral villages, with deaths along the way.[5] Restricting access to other medical care for prolonged periods led to higher rates of maternal and infant mortality in low- and middle-income countries worldwide.[6] And the economy is directly linked to public health, as the World Bank concluded when summarizing the connections between pandemic-related poverty and high rates of mortality for children under five.[7] As discussed in the introduction, the number of children living in multidimensional poverty massively increased in both 2020 and 2021.

The concept of focusing on resources before mass restrictions means providing adequate resources to improve living and working conditions so as to minimize the transmission of a virus. Since in the United States essential workers and those who could not work remotely were still asked to go to work, the resources we would need to provide include salary during times of isolation or quarantine; provision of safe isolation spaces; occupational health support, including well-fitting N95 masks and adequate workplace ventilation; core employment benefits such as paid sick leave; financial support for families of those who need to isolate; testing centers established in places where people live and work; and provision of universal healthcare coverage.

DO MORE FOR THOSE WHO NEED MORE

The second principle of our piece was: *do more for those who need more*. When in the fall of 2022 the CDC issued guidance that widespread universal masking was no longer necessary, that was perceived by some in the United States as a deep betrayal of equity. The pandemic had taken a disproportionate toll on racial/ethnic minorities prior to the distribution and increased uptake of vaccines, so the perception here was that continued universal masking could address inequities. However, embedded structural inequities cannot be fixed by a piece of cloth or a surgical mask made of polypropylene material. Fixing inequities is hard work and requires a true commitment to the concept of treating vulnerable populations in safety-net settings such as hospitals that treat publicly insured patients; equitable testing and vaccine distribution; aid to those who cannot work remotely; and resources to allow people who are ill to stay home without risking job loss or fearing that lost income will mean that bills can't be paid and food can't be bought.

Making sure that socioeconomic determinants of health are equitably distributed will require a commitment to combatting poverty, repairing our public education system, working on housing inequalities, and expanding access to healthcare. None of this can be fixed simply by imposing blanket mask mandates on the American public.

MEETING PEOPLE WHERE THEY ARE

The third principle we discussed in our *BMJ* blog piece is also a key element of the principle of harm reduction (which I'll discuss at the end of this chapter): *meeting people where they are.* By August 2022, when the CDC relaxed most of its suggested COVID-19 restrictions due to high levels of population immunity, a poll done by the *New York Times* revealed that most Americans were less worried about the virus than they had been and were getting back to normal life.[8] However, some public health officials did not take the pulse of the public into account before taking to social media and declaring that restrictions should be continued. As I've said several times in this book, COVID-19 will unfortunately never be over, and so we will require ongoing vaccination and application of therapeutics to deal with the virus. My life as an infectious diseases physician has been irrevocably altered by COVID-19, but I do think that public life can go back to normal when we have adequate biomedical interventions to combat COVID-19 (e.g., vaccines as well as oral antivirals for older people and the immunocompromised).[9] The analogy with HIV may be helpful here: we encouraged those living with HIV to know they would have a normal life (and life span) as our treatment and preventative tools expanded. Applying biomedical advances to an infectious disease while still taking the overall needs of individuals, public health, and society into account is how we managed the HIV epidemic.

Public health is a service industry, not a police force. Individuals should be able to decide for themselves how much they are willing to give up in order to avoid the risks of a respiratory pathogen. They should not be shamed or stigmatized by public health workers for wanting to visit a loved one in the hospital; for wanting to hold a funeral for their family member; for wanting to go to religious services; or for wanting to be around friends and family during holidays.[10]

The job of public health is to counsel people on how to stay safe. With HIV, for example, we initially counseled people to use condoms for HIV prevention, but we didn't tell people to forgo sexual intimacy. In the context of COVID-19, public health authorities seem to have forgotten some of these principles of harm reduction.[11] A survey from the United Kingdom conducted in September 2022 showed that only 1 percent of Britons were concerned about COVID-19 at that point, given the massive reductions in mortality brought about by vaccines and immunity.[12] However, the US media continued to publish pieces regarding how to stay safe during the holidays as late as October 2022, which may have led the public to think that our widely available vaccines weren't effective.[13]

PUBLIC HEALTH MUST BE DRIVEN BY DATA

The fourth principle my coauthors and I discussed was a call to revisit safety precautions as new data emerges. In the beginning precaution is fine, but eventually *public health must be driven by data*. I do believe that at the beginning of the pandemic lockdowns were a good idea, allowing us to figure out how this particular virus spread. I equate this to closing bathhouses in San Francisco and New York City at the beginning of HIV until we figured out ways to message about how to stay safe from HIV (with condoms at first and biomedical prevention tools later on). But lockdowns should be short, lasting only until we can put other mitigation procedures into place. When public health authorities are making decisions that affect people as profoundly as closures do, precaution should not be an absolute or indefinite mandate; rather, precaution should be a renewable contract.

As new information emerges, precautions should be revisited and altered quickly. For example, temperature screening, use of plexiglass shields, outdoor mask-wearing, school closures, beach closures, and prohibitions of outside gatherings are all examples of interventions that did not change the trajectory of the pandemic and should have been revisited more quickly. As discussed in Chapter 2, we can certainly recommend well-fitted, high-quality masks (such as N95, KN95, FFP2, and KF94 masks) for vulnerable individuals to help protect them against respiratory pathogens. But blanket mask mandates for entire populations didn't have good enough evidence behind them for public health officials to keep on imposing them, especially after vaccines were made available.

DEBATE AND DIALOGUE

Highly trained and knowledgeable professionals can interpret the same data in different ways. The only way to reconcile those different interpretations is through *debate and dialogue,* the fifth principle of public health.

We used to encourage medical and other professionals to engage in debate and dialogue as part of the process of tackling a complex problem like COVID-19, but during this pandemic debate was often stifled. For instance, mainstream media in the United States did report on the massive learning losses experienced by American children due to prolonged school closures and disruptions but did not report simultaneously that Sweden minimized school closures and that Swedish children did not undergo sustained learning loss.[14] The World Health Organization did not recommend masking young children five and under, but the CDC did, and American parents noticed the CDC's obvious deviation from WHO policy. Debate on social media or in articles regarding the effectiveness of masking at a population level (versus the effectiveness of masking for an individual) or the negative effects of lockdowns was often stifled and met with derision from other professionals.[15] Proposals regarding school openings in the United States—even though schools had opened much earlier in Europe and the United Kingdom—were often met with accusations of "wanting to kill children," which put a damper on discussion.

Engaging in debate regarding different approaches to a pandemic can result in a healthy middle ground and help lead us to more effective pandemic responses the next time.

DUTY AND SACRIFICE

Our sixth principle, *duty and sacrifice,* summarizes what public health professionals and doctors owe the world. First and foremost, we have a duty to our patients. For instance, there were doctors who declined to treat patients with HIV at the beginning of the HIV pandemic due to a fear of being infected. And many public health departments told hospitals and clinics to close down non-COVID-related medical care at the beginning of the pandemic. But closing down care for other medical conditions has consequences across the board, as seen in how cancer care, cardiovascular care, obstetric care, and care for other infectious diseases suffered.

For instance, since HIV is close to my heart, I was very concerned when UNAIDS put out a devastating report in July 2022 about setbacks to the HIV response during COVID.[16] Overall, the number of people living with HIV in the world has increased to 38.4 million, which is the highest number ever recorded. One of the most striking statistics is that approximately 1.5 million new HIV infections occurred in 2021—over 1 million more than the previously established UNAIDS global targets. In terms of treatment and mortality, 650,000 people died from AIDS-related illnesses in 2021, and only 28.7 million people out of the 38.4 million infected (75 percent) had access to antiretroviral therapy in 2021, leaving 25 percent, tragically, without access. Moreover, there were disparities in that access: 76 percent of adults age fifteen and older living with HIV had access to treatment, while only 52 percent of children had access.

The clinic I direct, Ward 86, is one of the oldest HIV clinics in the country. We were asked to shut down in-person care by the city and county of San Francisco on March 17, 2020. However, we could not close down in-person services for homeless patients, as many did not have access to telephones or stable places from which to participate in care via telehealth. We therefore remained open for them and quickly pivoted back to in-person care for all our patients when we saw rates of virologic suppression (the goal of HIV therapy for people living with HIV) drop in the spring and early summer of 2020.[17] We kept our staff safe with masks, distancing, and ventilation and had no COVID-19 transmissions among staff or patients in the clinic when seeing our patients in person. As a result of this resumption in care, we saw an increase in virologic suppression rates at Ward 86.[18] It is our duty to serve our patients and—despite not being in line with the ultra-precautionary principles set out by the San Francisco Department of Public Health (which did not pivot back to in-person care as quickly as we did)—the Ward 86 clinic fulfilled its duty to our patients during COVID-19.

Another aspect of this principle that's worth mentioning briefly is that public health and medical professionals should not benefit financially from the pandemic, including by collecting consulting fees, as doing so could be considered a conflict of interest. Yet during the COVID-19 response, some public health officials took consulting fees from pharmaceutical companies or from companies working on home delivery of goods.

SPEAKING TRUTH TO POWER

The seventh principle of public health is *speaking truth to power*. As I've mentioned earlier, some people were told they were "bad" if they caught COVID-19, especially if they had gathered with others. My coauthors and I felt strongly that shame-based messaging has no role in public health, and we felt an obligation to say so.

Shaming and stigmatizing people about an infection—or using pat phrases without nuance, like "just stay home" or "wear a mask; save lives"—did not take into account the structural constraints that forced many essential workers to take risks that other, more affluent individuals could avoid. The failure to recognize how such structural factors, including systemic racism and a failure to provide resources over restrictions, increased the risks of COVID-19 for some and not others is antithetical to public health, and we have an obligation to speak that truth loud and clear.

SPECIFIED INTERVENTIONS WITHOUT JUDGMENT

The eighth principle of public health we mentioned in our *BMJ* blog piece was *recommending interventions without judgment or undue enforcement*. Historically, and particularly during most of the HIV epidemic, public health's goal has been to disrupt normal life as little as possible while still preserving safety. Public health does not seek to massively alter the way of life of the populations it serves, which is why public health practitioners did not tell gay men to avoid sex altogether in order to prevent the spread of HIV or Mpox.[19] Rather, public health provides populations with guidance on how to stay safe, without judging or shaming people for the desires of the body or spirit, such as being with loved ones.[20] Studies performed during the HIV pandemic showed that providing empowering information on how to stay safe worked better than demanding abstinence-only approaches to HIV risk reduction.[21] The same would hold true for COVID-19.

PUBLIC HEALTH DOES NOT KNOW BORDERS

As we will discuss in Chapter 6, inequitable distribution of COVID-19 vaccines and therapeutics around the world resembled the inequities in the distribution of HIV treatments. But the ninth principle is that *public health does not know borders*. All public health is both local and global. Patents should not hold sway during a global public health emergency.

Moreover, we tried closing borders once different SARS-CoV-2 variants started to emerge, but that did not meaningfully prevent the transmission of infection.[22] South Africa—whose public health system was the first to describe the omicron variant—was "rewarded" for its careful work and transparent messaging with travel bans instituted by many Western countries, which very understandably upset African leaders.[23]

It's important here to add a word about closing borders to unvaccinated travelers. When the first COVID vaccines were rolled out, they initially were effective in almost completely blocking transmission of the alpha variant, which was the dominant strain at the time. However, as we've seen, the antibodies generated by the vaccine (and especially the antibodies that took up residence in the nose and throat) waned with time and were not as effective against later variants. During the omicron surge, both the vaccine and having had a previous infection made it about 21 percent less likely that someone with a breakthrough infection or a reinfection would pass the virus on to others (and those who had had both the vaccine and a previous infection were about 42 percent less likely to pass the virus on from a subsequent infection).[24] Therefore, banning people from entering a country based on vaccination status (as of the time of writing, the United States still prohibits unvaccinated noncitizens from entering the country) no longer makes sense.[25]

HARM REDUCTION

The last principle of public health that we discussed in our piece was *harm reduction*. As stated earlier, harm reduction—when applied to disease prevention, including for infectious diseases—is the principle of advising individuals how to mitigate risk, while acknowledging the real-world human desires or conditions that may lead individuals to take some risks. The goal of harm reduction is similar to the goal of lockdowns: reducing infections. However, harm-reduction-based approaches acknowledge and integrate realistic, pragmatic strategies that are responsive to the needs (financial and social) of human beings.

In the United States, the debates on COVID-19 strategies have increasingly been tied to political parties. Restrictions on businesses, limits on people's movement, and the use of non-pharmaceutical interventions such as mask mandates were seen as markers of being on the political left. People then attached varying moral dimensions to those interventions. However, while those on the political left also see public education as a universal good, it was precisely that group that tended to abandon that principle in the United States during COVID-19 with their advocacy of school closures.

While politics may contextualize public health, not every decision in public health can or should be viewed through a political lens. I am leftist in my politics, but I cannot see the prolonged school closures and the school disruptions in mainly Democratic-led states during COVID-19 as anything but politically motivated and harmful for the future health and prosperity of low-income children in the United States.[26]

My coauthors and I ended our piece in the *BMJ* blog with this statement, and I want to repeat it here:

The world continues to be more connected, facilitating both the best and worst of human experiences. From the perspective of infectious disease pandemics, it means that the emergence of a highly transmissible virus runs the risk of rapid global spread. Pandemic preparedness is more than data aggregators and rapid vaccine development, it is about leveraging the best of public health principles to support evidence-based and human-rights affirming responses to serve all, not just the wealthy.

CHAPTER 5

School Closures
and COVID-19

S ince the establishment of public education, policies surrounding the closure of schools due to pandemics or local epidemics have varied quite a bit. These policies remain contentious despite the many infectious disease outbreaks the world has encountered, because the data on what types of school closures should be implemented, under what conditions they should be in effect, and how long these closures should last have not been well aggregated. As a result, school closure policies have traditionally depended on existing public health practices, pandemic playbooks, and public expectations of the government's response at the local and national levels.[1]

SCHOOL CLOSURES DURING PREVIOUS INFECTIOUS DISEASE EPIDEMICS AND PANDEMICS

Comparing municipalities that did and did not close schools historically during pandemics does not clearly show a benefit in terms of disease trajectories. For example, during the 1918 influenza epidemic, many schools in the United States were closed for various lengths of time from September 1918 to January 1919. Amid widespread school closures, Dr. Royal S. Copeland and Dr. Sara Josephine Baker, who led the 1918 pandemic public health efforts in New York City, decided to keep schools open in their city. They reasoned that children were better off at school, where cleanliness was standardized and children had access to a school medical team that could quickly identify if they became sick. Furthermore, since three-quarters of the children in the public school system at the time lived in low-income housing, children needed access to vital services provided by these institutions, including nutrition and observation for neglect.[2] In comparison to the nearby cities of Boston and Philadelphia, both of which closed schools in September and October 1918, New York City's overall excess death rate during the 1918 pandemic (the number of deaths beyond the expected amount during the same season in a typical year) was actually lower.[3]

Even in a retrospective study that identified school closure as potentially having an impact on the excess death rate during the 1918 pandemic, the effect size of the intervention (that is, whether the impact of the intervention on the excess death rate is large or small) could not be determined.[4] Additionally, the study could not untangle the effects of other non-pharmaceutical interventions, such as isolation and quarantine, from those of school closure. Simply put, a rigorous evaluation of the historical precedent of school closures still has not uncovered whether school closures will make a substantial difference in the trajectory of a respiratory virus pandemic. Because of this, extended school closures have not been part of any previous pandemic playbook.

Since 1918, there have been many attempts, via modeling and observational studies, to better quantify the impact of short-term school closures on influenza-like illnesses, which have high transmission rates among children.[5] Results from these studies vary, however, with estimates of reduction in disease incidence and transmission ranging anywhere from 1 percent to 100 percent—a range so wide it's like doing no studies at all.[6]

Policies regarding schools during COVID also varied. However, unlike in previous pandemics, the extent of school closures for in-person learning, whether full or partial, was massive. For the thirteen months between March 2020 and June 2021, approximately 62 million US public school children were physically out of school.[7] During that time, on sixty-five days when there should have been school, students had no interactions whatsoever with teachers or peers—in other words, no school instruction on designated school time.[8] According to UNESCO, by March 2022, US schools had offered only partial in-person learning for over seventy weeks.[9]

While it's clear that school closures during COVID were far broader and longer than closures during previous pandemics in the United States, that raises a question: Was there something about COVID that made it different from previous pandemics and, therefore, made the extended closure of schools to in-person learning a reasonable measure?

ON THE NECESSITY OF EXTENDED SCHOOL CLOSURES

When the WHO declared a pandemic in March 2020, it was necessary for schools to shut down temporarily. This initial shutdown provided time for public health practitioners and government agencies to assess the epidemiology of the virus, including its transmission modalities and how to mitigate spread. More importantly, information on the severity of COVID in children and its transmissibility from children, both at school and in the home, was needed to chart a path toward school reopening. The answers to these questions began to emerge early on in the pandemic.

Children infected with COVID can exhibit no symptoms at all; several mild symptoms, including fever, dry cough, runny nose, congestion, and diarrhea; or severe symptoms that require mechanical ventilation support in the intensive care unit. Children can also develop a condition called multisystem inflammatory syndrome in children, or MIS-C. Patients with MIS-C typically exhibit a fever that lasts for three days or more and systemic, multiorgan symptoms such as rash, heart and blood vessel inflammation, and gastrointestinal symptoms.

By April 2020, researchers from the University of Pavia in Italy were able to identify eighteen studies coming out of China and Singapore in the preceding few months that provided the first clues to the severity of COVID-19 in children.[10] These studies detailed clinical outcomes in 1,065 patients under age nineteen. One infant who had severe COVID recovered with ICU support, and one death was documented in the age range ten to nineteen, though no other information was provided on the events that led up to that patient's death. The remaining patients experienced mild COVID and fully recovered within one to two weeks.

In June 2020, European members of the Pediatric Tuberculosis Trials Group published a study of the outcomes in 582 pediatric COVID-19 cases from eighty-two healthcare institutions across twenty-five European countries.[11] Among these cases, seventy-five patients (13 percent) required oxygen support, and four deaths were reported (0.7 percent); two of the patients with fatal outcomes were above the age of ten and had known preexisting conditions. Reassuringly, 87 percent of the children in the study did not require any respiratory support during their stay even though they were admitted to hospital settings.

These initial observations that COVID poses low risks of severe sequelae and fatality in children were further confirmed in a study by researchers collaborating across various major UK institutions in June 2021.[12] In this study, the authors used a mortality dataset linked to the UK hospital system and national COVID testing data, together with clinical review, to estimate the true severity of COVID in children. Out of 3,105 children who died between March 2020 and February 2021 in the United Kingdom, twenty-five died directly from COVID. When this number is divided by the total number of children and young people who tested positive for COVID in the United Kingdom during this same period, the infection fatality rate of COVID for children (that is, the percentage of children who die from COVID out of all children who tested positive for the condition) is 0.005 percent. An updated analysis over the first two years of the pandemic in the United Kingdom, as discussed in Chapter 2, demonstrated an infection fatality rate of 0.70/100,000 infections (0.0007 percent).[13] This rate contrasts sharply with the 1 percent mortality rate among adults over fifty prior to vaccines in the United Kingdom. It's notable that only some comorbidities seemed to result in death for children who developed COVID; while congenital heart conditions, obesity, cancer, and prematurity were some of the comorbid conditions in children who died from COVID, there were no deaths among infected children who also had isolated respiratory conditions (asthma, cystic fibrosis, etc.), type 1 diabetes, Down syndrome, or an isolated epilepsy diagnosis.[14]

While these studies showed that children do not tend to have severe acute cases of COVID, it was important in the calculus of school reopening to understand if there are long-term aftereffects for children who may initially have mild COVID cases. Fortunately, the most feared long-term effects are generally rare and manageable.[15] For example, MIS-C, which can develop several weeks after COVID, was seen in 0.03 percent of children who had COVID early in the pandemic.[16] MIS-C is also treatable, and the incidence of this condition has gone down even more over time, likely due to increasing population immunity.[17] Some children are reported to have developed PASC (long COVID), in which symptoms associated with COVID, such as headache and fatigue, last much longer than the period when patients test positive for the virus. In a study from the United Kingdom, surveillance data from 1,734 schoolchildren showed that COVID-related illness in most children lasts only six days.[18] For those whose symptoms lasted beyond twenty-eight days, most saw their symptoms resolve by around fifty-six days, or approximately eight weeks. Fortunately, the incidence of long COVID or PASC in children reported by these and other well-done studies (which included control groups of children who never had COVID) seems to be very low (much less than 1 percent) when the studies include control groups.[19]

Another long-term effect of COVID that caught the public's attention is the potential to develop heart and vascular conditions post-infection. A study from the United Kingdom puts this concern to rest when it comes to mild infection. In this study, the heart and vascular functions of seventy-four participants with confirmed mild COVID infections were compared to the functions of seventy-five participants who were confirmed (through lack of COVID nucleo-capsid antibodies) to have never had an infection.[20] Function tests were performed on these individuals anywhere between nine days and six months post-infection. There was no evidence of heart and vascular function differences between the study participants who had COVID and those who had not been infected. Moreover, the investigators in this study were blinded to the COVID-19 status of the individuals examined, eliminating potential bias. This bodes well for children who contract COVID-19, given that most infec-tions in children are mild.[21]

Knowing that most children who contract COVID have fa-vorable outcomes and low risks of long-term sequelae, even in cases where they have underlying health conditions, the next is-sue to address is whether children are the main driver of COVID transmission in their schools and communities. One of the earli-est comprehensive studies to address transmissibility of COVID in children came from the European Centre for Disease Prevention and Control (ECDC) in August 2020.[22] In this study, fifteen Eu-ropean countries were surveyed for COVID outbreaks that may have been related to schools. Most schools in this study did not report any outbreaks, even when the schools were in session. Of those that reported outbreaks, the number of individuals associated with a school outbreak was typically very small, with ten people in an outbreak cluster being an exceptionally large number. Based on this information, the ECDC concluded that schools are not places where COVID tends to substantially spread.

The ECDC then followed up with ongoing surveys and literature reviews of the transmission rate of COVID-19 between children and from children to adults.[23] Studies from Germany, France, Ireland, Finland, Australia, Singapore, the United States, and Israel all suggested that transmission between children in schools is uncommon: if children do exhibit COVID symptoms at the same time as school reopening, the case was less likely to be from school and more likely to have been acquired in the community. In studies from Australia, Ireland, and the Netherlands, children were not identified as the primary driver of adult COVID cases in schools.

This initial observation from the ECDC that COVID transmission is not driven by children in schools was further confirmed by later studies from other countries. A German study of 2,500 parent-child pairs, with children being between the ages of five and ten, aimed to determine the prevalence of COVID in children and adults during a period of lockdown.[24] The study also asked whether children who needed to attend daycare facilities had a higher risk of developing COVID compared to those who did not attend these facilities. The results show that overall, the prevalence of COVID in children was one-third lower than in adults, suggesting that children are not the primary driver of COVID outbreaks. There was also no evidence that children who attended daycare facilities had any higher risk of contracting COVID compared to those who stayed at home. This was an important finding, as children in daycare facilities likely could not maintain the consistent hygiene practices recommended for the prevention of COVID spread, such as masking and social distancing.

Subsequent to the publication of this study, several other studies reached the same conclusions: (1) that children in school were not the primary driver of COVID transmission, as they had lower rates of COVID positivity compared to the adults in school; (2) that COVID transmission in schools was driven by adult staff members, who acquired COVID from the community and brought the infection into school; and (3) that even though COVID did spread in schools, the incidence of COVID in schools remained consistently lower than the incidence of COVID in the community, with one study estimating that school incidence was 37 percent lower than community incidence during the same time frame.[25] These studies were conducted in age groups ranging from children in daycare all the way through high school, indicating that the epidemiology of COVID is consistent in children under eighteen.

Additionally, while these studies could provide some detail on COVID transmission from and to children, it was more difficult to assess what mitigation strategies might be needed to slow transmission within schools. In most of the studies, masking was required in schools. Some schools had additional social distancing (with the required distance varying from three feet to six feet) and grouping protocols to try to decrease COVID spread; in other schools this was not feasible due to space and resource availability.[26] Some schools had a community spread threshold for school reopening, while others did not.[27] These studies also did not include control groups (groups where masking and hygiene interventions were not implemented for comparison). That's why researchers find it hard to determine if these extra measures made a difference in containing COVID within schools.

However, the fact that hygiene measures were implemented differently in the different schools studied but the conclusions from the studies remain the same provides strong supporting evidence that staff and students were safe in school during COVID, even before the vaccines were introduced and regardless of the hygiene measures taken. The low rates of transmission in school settings from studies conducted in the United States across a variety of settings—Wisconsin, North Carolina, Utah, and New York City—were well documented.[28] Furthermore, by April 2021, nearly 80 percent of teachers had received at least one dose of a COVID vaccine.[29] This made schools an even safer environment for all members of the school community, especially because adults are the primary drivers of COVID spread, vaccines work well to prevent severe disease and death regardless of the variant, and vaccination of some members in a community provides partial protection against COVID for individuals who cannot yet get vaccinated.[30] Based on all this information, I wrote multiple pieces with other public health experts on why schools should be reopened once vaccines were available for teachers.[31]

If, overall, COVID infections in children are mostly mild, with severe long-term sequelae uncommon, and if the spread of COVID is not driven by schools, that brings us back to the question we raised at the beginning of this chapter: Was there something about COVID that was different from previous pandemics and thereby justified the extended school closures?

To answer this question, let's take a closer look at the largest respiratory pandemic in modern times, the 1918 influenza. As previously mentioned, when the 1918 pandemic began to sweep across the United States, many states and localities did decide to close schools, though the median length of school closure was only thirty-six days, and the maximum length was ninety days.[32] The extended school closures for in-person learning seen during COVID-19 would make sense if at its height COVID-19 posed more of a danger to children than the 1918 influenza pandemic posed at its peak. However, the opposite is true. Using US data, we find that the 1918 pandemic saw a high mortality rate for young people: 10 out of every 1,000 infants died of that flu, and 2 out of every 1,000 children aged five to fifteen died.[33] In contrast, the mortality rate for COVID was just 0.0003 deaths per 1,000 infants and 0.0002 deaths for every 1,000 children between five and fourteen.[34]

When the test of historical precedent fails, we must next look to the responses of countries similar to the United States during COVID-19 and ask if the measures employed for US schools during the pandemic are comparable. Using data from UNESCO, the United States appears to be an outlier among other high-income countries, keeping schools fully open for in-person learning only 13 percent of the time from February 2020 to March 2022.[35] Having the lowest rate of full in-person schooling among high-income countries did not seem to help the United States with its COVID mortality rates—data from Johns Hopkins shows that the United States had a higher mortality rate than at least nine other high-income countries that kept their schools open at least 50 percent of the time.[36] Together, these results lead us to the conclusion that the extended school closures in the United States were not only unprecedented but also unnecessary and unjustified.

WHAT HAPPENED IN THE UNITED STATES?

One factor leading to this disastrous policy failure in the United States was that public health authorities and medical doctors are often Democrats, and this is reflected in the policies that were put in place during the pandemic.[37] Indeed, blue states exhibited more prolonged school closures and disruptions than did red states, and school openings and education became associated with the Republican Party, with the Republican president at the time pushing for school reopenings as early as the summer of 2020.[38]

Another reason was the strong negative bias of COVID news coverage in the United States, even after vaccines had become widely available. In one study, 20,000 English-language COVID news articles were analyzed for their tone. The researchers discovered that, compared to other countries' COVID coverage and general US media coverage of other topics, the top fifteen US news outlets were 25 percent more likely to cover any development related to COVID, whether good or bad, in a negative tone. For instance, stories of increasing COVID-19 cases outnumbered stories of decreasing cases by a factor of 5.5, even during periods when new cases were declining. The report noted that the "negativity of the U.S. major media is notable even in areas with positive scientific developments including school re-openings and vaccine trials."[39] The rate of negative coverage remained high regardless of the political leanings of the news outlets' audience. And that negativity didn't seem to be affected by the actual trajectory of the pandemic as measured by case and hospitalization numbers.

It is one thing for news coverage to be negative and accurate. However, much negative coverage of COVID relied on inaccurate initial modeling data and misinterpretation of publicly available information.[40] This phenomenon was most prominently exemplified by the news coverage surrounding the spread of B.1.1.7 (the alpha variant) by children. In March 2021, reports coming out of Michigan stated that this new variant seemed to be spreading more rapidly in and through children, leading to a higher increase in overall COVID hospitalizations for the state and justifying the need for schools to resume virtual learning.[41] What those reports failed to mention is that the number of weekly cases in school-age Michigan children (under nineteen years of age) was usually still lower than the number for middle-aged adults, who had full access to vaccines by that point in the pandemic.[42] Therefore, children were not likely the primary driver for the spread of the alpha variant and increased hospitalizations in Michigan in early 2021.

The news narrative that COVID was deadlier to children than the flu (that is, recent flu strains, not the 1918 pandemic strain) also exerted pressure on schools to continue being remote.[43] Some argued that because fewer children were sick with the flu compared to COVID and because those who became sick with the flu had fewer problematic sequelae than kids who contracted COVID, extended remote learning was a necessary measure. But this is false, and for a simple reason: at no point in history have we ever tested children for influenza as we have tested for COVID. Usually when children exhibit flu symptoms, they are taken to the doctor's office to receive an antigen test that confirms their positive status. For COVID, children are frequently tested in school and hospital settings regardless of symptoms or lack thereof.[44] This makes comparing the two conditions for prevalence and severity virtually impossible. Furthermore, the results of these comparisons often conflate children who die *from* COVID, which is an important measure in understanding the severity of this single condition in children, with children who happen to have died *with* COVID, even if the virus did not contribute to their death or hospitalization.[45]

A third factor was inaccurate modeling. From the beginning of the pandemic, models that turned out to be inaccurate informed a significant amount of US policy. In turn, school administrators, legislators, and governors frequently cited such policy in their own decisions regarding prolonged school closures.[46] In January 2021, for example, a biostatistician modeler serving as a consultant to a large school district in Oregon gave a presentation to a widely attended public school board meeting. His model predicted that COVID-19 hospitalizations in Oregon would nearly double in February and March of that year, based on assumptions about variants and people's fatigue with mitigation measures.[47] Note that this model was constructed at a time when vaccine rollout for adults in the state was brisk.

In a video of the meeting, school board members can be seen asking fearful questions about this grim scenario. One board member comments, "My fear is we are going to get both the fatigue and the variant."[48] Yet between January and March, hospitalizations in the region *fell* by 66 percent.[49] This school district maintained fully remote learning into April 2021, despite some of the lowest

COVID-19 rates in the country.[50] Even when in-person instruction resumed, however, elementary school children were back initially for only two and a half hours a day, four days per week.[51] Furthermore, while the severity of COVID in children and their influence on the spread of COVID were exaggerated, mental health concerns in children were selectively downplayed, contributing to the public perception that remote learning could be continued.

Another significant factor was public rhetoric that, sadly and inaccurately, pitted those who wanted schools reopened against those who wanted to save lives. Fueling this rhetoric was misinformation promoted by media outlets, which gave a platform to experts who were fitting the data to preconceived narratives rather than trying to determine what narrative most accurately fit the data we had. Both large and small media outlets routinely amplified voices of COVID-19 experts with large social media platforms without vetting or correcting their claims; however, large media outlets have data bureaus that could and should have investigated these claims, using publicly available data, before amplifying them. Many of these experts touted the public health benefits of school closures, even though that policy was not supported by the data and underplayed the academic, social-emotional, and health costs such closures imposed on students, families, and society as a whole.

A DISASTROUS POLICY

In March 2020, Dr. Jennifer Nuzzo (now at the Brown School of Public Health) wrote an op-ed warning that a measure as drastic as school closure would have heavy unintended consequences for society.[52] For example, she said, parents might need to quit their jobs to stay home and watch their children, something that would disproportionally affect poor communities and women. Additionally, social services programs that ensure students have nutritious food and a safe place for after-school activities would be disrupted. Education interruptions could further exacerbate the achievement gap between students from high-income families and those from low-income families.

Following the publication of Nuzzo's piece, experts from various institutions in the United States, the United Kingdom, Italy, and Hong Kong similarly warned of such unintended consequences. The potential for learning loss induced by school closures was a consistent theme across all these pieces, especially when roughly 4–5 percent of children in high-income countries like the United Kingdom and the United States still have no access to stable internet connections and safe home conditions for studying.[53]

Children tend to gain more weight during times of school breaks, and so some experts were worried that extended school closures could lead to unhealthy weight gain among children—which was recorded two years later.[54] In addition to physical health concerns, mental well-being has been documented to decrease during extended summer breaks, making children's mental health another reason to worry about school closures.[55] A third concern was that with schools closing to in-person instruction, domestic violence, child abuse, and neglect could rise but go unreported. This concern was reinforced by the experience of the Ebola outbreak in West Africa from 2014 to 2016, where the closure of schools for five months led to increased rates of sexual abuse and exploitation. Teenage pregnancies also doubled in Sierra Leone during this time.[56]

Two months into the COVID-19 pandemic, these warnings began to manifest into reality. In May 2020, doctors at John Muir Medical Center in Walnut Creek, California, reported that they were seeing more cases of deaths by suicide than deaths by COVID, particularly among young adults. The head of the Trauma Department at John Muir said: "We've never seen numbers like this, in such a short period of time. I mean we've seen a year's worth of suicide attempts in the last four weeks."[57]

By the end of 2020, the anecdotal evidence provided by health centers across the United States began to be codified in official reports. In November 2020, the CDC published an analysis of the rate of pediatric mental health emergency department (ED) visits from January to October 2020.[58] The data showed that while the number of pediatric ED visits decreased overall, the proportion of these visits made up by mental health visits had increased relative to 2019. At this stage in the pandemic, one hypothesis that could be inferred from this study is that mental health struggles were starting to bubble up in children, but public health messages warning the public not to use the ED unless absolutely needed (to save resources for fighting COVID) could have decreased the overall number of ED visits. Parents who took their children to the ED must have noted problems serious enough to disregard these warnings.

This hypothesis was later proven to be correct when the CDC published a follow-up report in June 2021.[59] The report uses pediatric ED visit data from January 2019 to May 2021 to show that while there were fewer ED visits for suspected suicide attempts from March to April 2020 compared to the same time in 2019, this number began to change in May 2020. Starting in that month, the average weekly number of ED visits for girls ages twelve to seventeen with suspected suicide attempts increased by 26.2 percent relative to May 2019. By the winter of 2020, this number climbed to 39.1 percent higher than for the same period in 2019. For young adults ages eighteen to twenty-five, overall attempted suicide rates in 2020 were between 1.1 and 1.6 times higher than in 2019. Independent reports of hospitals around the United States—including Children's Hospital Colorado, emergency departments in Connecticut, and hospitals in the Boston area—not having enough beds for children with mental health needs provide further evidence that by the middle of 2021, the substantial harms of unnecessary school closure in 2020 had come to a head.[60]

The mental health crisis among children continued to worsen as the pandemic went on. A CDC report estimated the rate of attempted suicide among girls as 50.6 percent higher during winter 2021 than winter 2019.[61] Suicide attempt rates also increased in boys, though only by 3.7 percent. One explanation is that females are known to have higher rates of suicide attempts, while males typically have higher rates of completed suicides.[62] This also suggests that early warning signs of a mental health crisis are probably best seen in the rate of mental health services utilization, not in rates of attempted or completed suicide. Data from California's Bay Area shows increased visits to emergency rooms for children in mental health crisis, increased suicidality, and a higher prevalence of eating disorders.[63] In any case, we should never have ignored signs of despair in our youth. Finally, on December 7, 2021, the US surgeon general sounded the alarm regarding the mental health crisis among our nation's youth.[64] By November 2022, the CDC cited data that showed three-quarters of children had experienced at least one adverse childhood event (ACE) related to the COVID-19 pandemic response, including abuse, neglect, witnessing violence, or having a family member attempt or die by suicide.[65]

School closures also caused many children to forgo necessary physical health screenings through school health programs or through teacher observations. For this reason, other health conditions in children, such as myopia, anorexia, and obesity, began to rise.[66] One unintended consequence of being hyperfocused on preventing COVID in children is of particular concern: children falling behind on their routine vaccination schedule. With in-person school, it was important and often mandated for children to be vaccinated for conditions such as measles, polio, whooping cough, and more. The lack of in-person schooling meant children were not being checked for routine vaccinations, leaving children more vulnerable to these diseases, which arguably are more dangerous to them than COVID. According to a report by UNICEF and WHO, over 25 million children worldwide missed out on essential vaccinations in 2020–2021; large measles outbreaks in Zimbabwe and India were consequently seen in 2022.[67] By November 2022, the United Nations reported that 40 million children worldwide were susceptible to measles due to COVID-19-related disruptions in care.[68]

In addition to the exacerbation of mental and physical health issues in children, experts warned that school closings could mean that child abuse would go unreported. One study published in October 2020 used the number of child abuse reports in the state of Florida from January 2006 to April 2020 to provide a conservative estimate of a 27 percent decrease in child abuse reports in the state during March and April 2020.[69] Applying this number nationwide, the researchers estimated that roughly 212,500 potential cases of child abuse were not reported, and because approximately 22 percent of all reported cases are confirmed, roughly 40,000 actual cases of abuse went undetected. Because teachers make most of the initial abuse reports, many of these undetected cases could likely be attributed to the closure of in-person schooling. By November 2022, in the country with the longest pandemic-related school closures (the Philippines), one of five children were reported to be subject to sexual exploitation.[70]

Academic learning loss is another aspect of school closures that will have profound health implications on this generation for years to come. Online learning was thought to be a sufficient replacement for in-person learning early in the pandemic. However, the high rate of children dropping out of school completely suggests that this massive experiment of extended online schooling for children can be deemed a failure. One estimate is that up to 3 million children in the United States—approximately the number of schoolchildren in the state of Florida—completely lost contact with schools during the pandemic.[71] The reasons include lack of access to stable internet service, children having increased burdens as primary caretakers in families where parents lost their jobs, and basic disinterest in online school.[72]

For children who did remain in school throughout the closures, the quality of their education declined drastically, as evidenced in the high rates of students failing their classes. In California—the US state with the lowest level of in-person instruction—some of the largest school districts saw the highest upticks in failing grades.[73] Some schools began to employ grade inflation to keep students on track for graduation. For example, in West Contra Costa Unified School District, students will only receive a grade of F if their final score is under 50 percent; traditionally, the threshold to receive a failing grade is 59 percent.[74] Other districts switched from a letter grade system to a pass/fail system, which unfortunately tends to make it harder for students to be motivated in school.

When California released standardized test results for the 2020–2021 school year, it became clear why schools were using grade adjustment measures to ensure that students could continue to the next grade or educational institution: only 49 percent of students assessed in grades 3–8 and grade 11 met or exceeded a grade-appropriate level of achievement in English; only 34 percent of students in the same grades achieved appropriate educational attainment in mathematics.[75] This is a decline from the already abysmal pre-pandemic figures of 51 percent having an appropriate level of achievement in English and 40 percent in math. And because many students completely stopped attending school during the pandemic, using percentages to assess the proportion of test-taking students who reached appropriate milestones likely provides a conservative estimate of learning loss, as those figures cannot account for students who simply were not in school.

For children with special educational needs, the loss of learning was demonstrated even earlier in the pandemic. In July 2020, a study from Iran showed that in a survey of 1,100 parents/caretakers, 39 percent reported that their children with special educational needs were struggling with cognitive, learning, and communication problems, and 61 percent reported that resources available to support them and their child disappeared during the pandemic.[76] Similar reports from the United States showed that students with disabilities, such as autism spectrum disorders, hearing deficits, and vision loss, also struggled with remote online learning.[77]

Learning loss in any community is concerning, but it is particularly concerning when it occurs in marginalized and poor communities. A report from June 2020 estimated that if schools were to return to in-person learning by January 2021—which did not happen in many blue states within the United States—low-income students would have lost 12.4 months of schooling in comparison to 6 months of learning lost by more affluent students.[78]

This learning loss is projected to have long-term effects on income as children grow up. Using the scenario described above (and remember, in some states students remained in remote learning for longer), on average, white students would be expected to see an income reduction of $1,348 per year over their adult working life because of the education loss. For Black students, the educational loss could translate to an income reduction of $2,186 per year as adults.[79] Over a lifetime of earning, the total losses are huge. One reason this matters is that wealth has consistently been shown to be a strong determinant of health outcomes and life expectancy.[80] Furthermore, education remains one of the most stable pathways out of poverty in the United States. When education opportunities are taken away from these communities, the cycle of poverty perpetuates, thus exacerbating health disparities that already existed pre-pandemic.

The pandemic and prolonged school closures that disrupted the lives of children and adolescents amplified the challenges facing America's youth, particularly among historically marginalized groups. With widespread school closures, many children were unable to effectively learn, interact in groups, engage, socialize, be active, eat healthy food, or get support. Children with special needs and from disadvantaged backgrounds in general paid a significant price. A report from the Center for Education Policy Research at Harvard University found that high-poverty schools both spent more weeks in remote instruction during 2020–2021 and suffered large losses in achievement when they did so.[81] Students in high-poverty schools did not often have parents home to coach them through online school or private places from which to take online instruction. The massive extent of the learning losses experienced by American children due to prolonged school closures and disruptions were reported by the National Assessment of Educational Progress in August 2022, showing clear disparities that most affected Black and Hispanic children.[82] Decades of work have attempted to close the racial and socioeconomic learning gaps in the United States, but the school closures and limited access to remote learning that disproportionately affected marginalized communities threaten to widen those gaps. In September 2022, major progressive media outlets in the United States finally began to call out school policy failures, the need for Democrats to reclaim the mantle of the "education party," and the massive learning losses sustained by our most vulnerable children due to the COVID response.[83]

The same trends in child harm have been seen globally, as many countries followed the US example in school closures, given the prominent role the United States has played in global health policy. UNICEF warned throughout the pandemic of the devastating impact on children of school closures and other aspects of COVID, highlighting child poverty, child health and mortality, learning loss, early girl marriage, child well-being, child malnutrition, routine childhood vaccination rates, effects of HIV, child violence, exploitation, and abuse.[84] Since early childhood education for girls is important for future women's empowerment, the effects of the devastating educational setbacks for girls during COVID may last a generation.[85] As UNICEF executive director Henrietta Fore stated, "The evidence is clear: prolonged, nationwide school closures, limited resources for students, teachers and parents and lack of access to remote learning have wiped out decades of progress in education and rendered childhood unrecognizable. A shadow pandemic of child labor, child marriage and mental health issues has taken hold."[86]

Given all the negative impacts that school closure had on children, it is surprising that this policy was pursued for so long. Even when more schools started to reopen for in-person learning in 2021–2022, continual disruptions—from weekly testing for asymptomatic low-risk children, quarantines, and mandatory masking (even after child vaccines were available)—made it harder for children to be at and remain in school.[87] Nearly half of the students in the Los Angeles Unified School District were chronically absent in

2021–2022.[88] Based on the associations between school disruptions, decreased educational attainment, and decreased life expectancy, one model estimated that missed primary school instruction during 2020 could be associated with a loss of life expectancy greater than would have been observed if leaving schools open had led to more deaths during the first wave of the pandemic (which, to reiterate, did not happen).[89]

DIFFERENCES IN SCHOOL POLICIES: UNITED STATES VERSUS UNITED KINGDOM AND EUROPE

Countries that began and maintained in-person teaching during rates of high community transmission did not see a sharp rise in cases, as feared by many in the US government. A report conducted by the Norwegian Institute of Public Health revealed that allowing schools in Norway to remain open did not lead to a spike in cases, and in fact most outbreaks were associated with transmission outside the school setting.[90] Another study in Norway sought to measure what's called the secondary attack rate, the likelihood that people associated with an infected individual become infected; in this case the researchers used other students and faculty in order to measure the spread within a school. Their work demonstrated that as long as schools maintained strict infection prevention and control measures, they were able to significantly limit the number of such secondary cases (in many cases no or only one other person was infected, and there was only a minuscule number of clusters).[91] A similar study conducted in Zurich indicated similar results, with almost half of these secondary infections presenting as asymptomatic.[92] This data is corroborated by additional large contact tracing studies done in Australia and South Korea, as well as a population-level study conducted in Italy.[93] Importantly, a study in Sweden demonstrated that teachers of younger students generally had lower rates of infection than those who taught older students. As younger students tend to be most vulnerable to the problems caused by online learning, this is a promising indication that maintaining in-person school is a viable option.[94] Not only do school openings not significantly increase transmission, but an analysis done in the United Kingdom indicated no additional likelihood of death from COVID-19 (and in some cases even a *reduced* likelihood of death) when adults under the age of sixty-five share a household with a school-going child up to eleven years old.[95]

While demonstrating low transmissibility within schools is important, it is also vital to understand whether keeping schools open leads to increased household transmission. This can help us understand whether children could be a potential driver of spread within older and more vulnerable populations, throwing a wrench into the viability of keeping schools open. However, a study conducted in Korea found that the secondary attack rate from children to household members was low as long as positive cases were handled with proper social distancing measures.[96]

In fact, even data from the United States found no evidence for secondary infection that would support prolonged school closures. A study using national US data demonstrated that while school openings may have been associated with higher case rates in some regions, primarily the South, this increase was not correlated strongly to increases in COVID-19 mortality.[97] And researchers at the Duke University School of Medicine and UNC–Chapel Hill did an analysis of fifty-six school districts in North Carolina that revealed very low transmission rates within schools that employed mitigation procedures.[98]

While many of these international studies provide evidence that closing schools during the COVID-19 pandemic produced at most only minimal benefit in terms of infection rates, additional studies sought to characterize the intrinsic value of reopening schools by measuring learning loss in countries other than the United States. An extremely comprehensive study analyzed data from Dutch primary schools from 2017 to 2020, with a sample size of approximately 350,000 students.[99] Specifically, the researchers investigated the difference in test scores across various demographics, including household education level, sex, school grade, subject, and prior performance. Their results indicated that students in the Netherlands experienced a drop of 3 percentile points in test scores across math, spelling, and reading—drops that correlated to the duration of school closure, which was relatively short in that country at approximately eight weeks. Even more concerning was data indicating that students from less-educated and underresourced households experienced a 50–60 percent increase in learning loss compared to students from more affluent households. These learning losses were certainly even greater in countries that had prolonged school lockdowns.

Other studies attempted to measure the intangible and psychosocial losses incurred by isolation. A Swedish study demonstrated that during the pandemic students experienced only minor decreases in self-esteem and perceived support from teachers and overall had no increase in the frequency of emotional or mental health issues.[100] The study authors attribute much of these results to Sweden's maintenance of in-person schooling and noted that a stable in-person learning environment led to resilience in children. In contrast, children around the world who remained in isolation experienced a dramatic loss in social and physical engagement and an increase in depression/anxiety, as determined by a large *Lancet* commission published in September 2022 on the world's pandemic response. (The *Lancet* is a prominent medical journal that often commissions pieces to evaluate policies and provide recommendations for pressing medical issues.)[101]

Unfortunately, these losses will have extremely tangible effects on students. The *Lancet* commission noted that the closure of schools in 195 countries affected almost 1.5 billion children worldwide, leading to deleterious effects ranging from socioemotional outcomes to increased levels of abuse.[102] Globally, they pointed out, girls especially suffered ill effects because of not receiving adequate care and protection. And the commission emphasized that school reopening was not appropriately prioritized in comparison to other activities.

As reported by the World Bank, UNICEF, and UNESCO in December 2021, across the globe the current generation of students now risks losing $17 trillion in lifetime earnings (about 14 percent of today's global GDP) as a result of COVID-19 pandemic-related school closures. This new projection reveals that the impact is more severe than previously thought, far exceeding the $10 trillion estimate released in 2020. The report shows that in low- and middle-income countries, the share of children living in "learning poverty" (defined as being "unable to read and understand a simple age-appropriate text at age 10")—already 53 percent before the pandemic—could potentially reach 70 percent given the long school closures and the ineffectiveness of remote learning for many students worldwide.[103]

The United Nations held an education summit on September 16, 2022, to discuss ways to combat the drastic learning losses worldwide from the COVID-19 pandemic.[104] UN secretary general António Guterres said that education worldwide was in "a deep crisis." "Instead of being the great enabler," he pointed out, education is fast becoming "a great divider." He highlighted data showing that some 70 percent of ten-year-olds in poor countries are unable to read and are "barely learning." The school closures during COVID-19 "dealt a hammer blow to progress on SDG4," the Sustainable Development Goal targeting equitable quality education.[105] The losses were particularly marked for girls, with increases in teenage pregnancies, abuse, learning loss (where sons' needs for remote learning were prioritized over daughters' needs), and sex work occurring during the pandemic.[106] The UN press release also noted that these losses will only continue to widen disparities unless countries significantly intervene and prioritize offsetting the losses suffered during these school closures.

UNICEF repeatedly warned during the pandemic that school closures were not necessary for COVID-19 pandemic control and would incur a great deal of collateral damage. On January 23,

2022, UNICEF reported that the scale of education loss during COVID-19 was "nearly insurmountable" and needed to be rectified immediately.[107] The UNICEF report details that more than 616 million students remained affected by full or partial school closures as of January 24, 2022 (the International Day of Education). UNICEF went over the data on learning loss in various countries, reporting that across Brazil one in ten students ages ten to fifteen were not planning to return to school once their schools reopened; that in South Africa schoolchildren were three-quarters to a full school year behind where they should be and that up to half a million students dropped out of school altogether; and that in the United States learning losses have been observed in many states, including Texas, California, Colorado, Tennessee, North Carolina, Ohio, Virginia, and Maryland.

As Robert Jenkins, UNICEF's chief of education, articulated the problem: "While the disruptions to learning must end, just reopening schools is not enough. Students need intensive support to recover lost education. Schools must also go beyond places of learning to rebuild children's mental and physical health, social development and nutrition." UNICEF reported at that time that over 370 million students had lost access to meals provided by school districts, only further exacerbating health disparities for low-income students.[108] This averages out to four of ten school meals being missed around the world, per the *Lancet* commission.[109] Beyond the loss of regular nutrition, the UNICEF report from January 2022 also discussed the impact on child abuse and children's mental health, noting high rates of anxiety and depression among children and young people, with some studies finding that girls, adolescents, and those living in rural areas are most likely to experience these mental health effects. As *The Economist* lamented in July 2022, COVID learning loss has been a global disaster, anticipated by some but surprising many.[110]

It becomes important, then, to understand the United States' rationale behind maintaining school closures when other countries moved to reopen schools. Anthony LaMesa, a freelance education consultant, argues that for one thing, the decentralized control of schools in the United States ultimately made it very difficult to coordinate a robust plan for reopening.[111] For another, in Europe many teachers advocated for altering the infrastructure of schools in order to make them safer during COVID, rather than simply arguing for or against closures. In response, many European schools invested in hiring a large number of teachers in order to reduce class size and to temporarily replace teachers who were medically vulnerable, and they installed better ventilation systems.

Perhaps the most sobering conclusion from all this data is that the US government failed to adequately prioritize the needs of American students. By being unwilling to consider the multiple losses that resulted from school closures, the United States ultimately failed in its duty to invest in its future generations. As the ECDC pointed out, school closures should be only a "last resort" because of the severe damage they can inflict on children.[112]

As a September 2022 *New Yorker* article on the value of returning to normalcy pointed out with regard to school closures:

> This was a trade off-we chose—mortgaging the quality of education in an effort to protect parents, teachers, communities, and (to a lesser extent) children themselves from the coronavirus.

> Now the U.S. seems to have arrived at another judgment: the value of normalcy exceeds that of caution.[113]

Starting now, we ought to do everything in our power to holistically prioritize the health, education, and development of our children.

MOVING FORWARD

It is impossible to go back in time and correct the damage done to our youth during COVID, but we can still try to prevent fear and negativity from having such a strong influence on policy decisions in future pandemics by taking six necessary steps.

First, any process of meaningful reform will require a formal inquiry or a commission to look into the United States' pandemic response, either through the government or through private initiatives. Other countries have conducted such inquiries (Norway, Sweden, the Netherlands, the United Kingdom, Denmark, and Australia) and made the results available to the public and to decision-makers.[114] All the assessments performed to date have concluded that schools should remain open as much as possible during crises in order to ensure that children get the education they need, receive support for their mental health, and avoid the future economic costs of present-day school closures.

Second, school decision-makers should stop relying on predictive models. Too often they are wrong and result in unnecessarily large (and harmful) degrees of caution when it comes to school reopening. Instead, modelers and media outlets should draw upon publicly available real-world data from the CDC and vetted state databases. They should avoid using inputs based on assumptions related to unquantifiable human behaviors, such as fear and fatigue, and instead construct their models using quantifiable data such as local hospitalization rates, in-school transmission events, and vaccination rates. One imperative for model creation after vaccines became available should have been to distinguish COVID-19 hospitalizations as being "with" or "for" COVID, since we continued to swab every patient being admitted to a US hospital for COVID, regardless of symptoms.[115] As I noted in Chapter 2, data from Massachusetts in the omicron era showed that the majority of hospitalizations were misclassified, with patients being listed as admitted *for* COVID when in fact they were being admitted for other reasons and also happened to test positive for COVID.[116] A chart review published in an infectious diseases journal in August 2022 confirmed that this misclassification occurs, and pointed out that it underestimates the power of vaccines.[117] That same month, the United Kingdom stopped the practice of testing asymptomatic individuals admitted to hospitals.[118] I believe that greater media coverage of immunology, explaining it to the public, could have helped quell some of the panic surrounding inaccurate COVID models.

Third, as I pointed out earlier in this chapter, much misinformation comes from experts fitting data to preconceived narratives rather than starting with the data and then trying to see what narrative best fits it. Although misinformation is difficult to stop, large media outlets have the ability to investigate these narratives before repeating and amplifying them. They should also ensure that in their reporting they are using best data practices, such as comparing case and hospitalization numbers corrected for population distribution.

Fourth, prior to the next pandemic, strategies should be put into place for determining under what conditions schools should close and switch to remote learning, what other non-pharmaceutical interventions need to be put into place in schools, and for how long the measures should exist. Even though we've had several major pandemics in the twentieth and twenty-first centuries, definitive answers to these questions are still not available. Cluster randomized trials, which would allow for clear understanding of cause and effect, should be utilized extensively to obtain accurate information on the efficacy and harm of non-pharmaceutical interventions.[119] This would ensure that we will not be choosing options that have well-documented harms but no benefits, as we have done throughout the COVID-19 pandemic when it comes to children.

Fifth, when it comes to issues affecting children, teachers have always been children's best advocates. However, since teaching is one of the lowest-paying jobs in the United States, many teachers often must spend their own money purchasing classroom supplies for their students, and cases of teachers being disrespected by students, parents, and school administrations are common.[120] All these factors contribute to burnout and to teachers' mistrust toward school administrations and parents, as evidenced in the massive rate of teachers leaving the profession—an exodus that was exacerbated by the stressors of the COVID pandemic.[121] Even when parents and school districts wanted to reopen schools for children, years of feeling devalued made it difficult for teachers to see that decision as being in the best interest of their profession as well. Therefore, being fully prepared for a pandemic requires significant investments not just in the infrastructure of public health and research but also in funding teachers adequately and rebuilding trust between teachers, parents, and the school system.

Sixth, as outlined by Dr. Leslie Bienen (of Oregon Health & Science University–Portland State University School of Public Health), we need to provide American children with a federally mandated right to an education.[122] It was not until 1918 that every state required children to go to school, and the US Department of Education was not established as a separate federal department until 1979. At this point, only some state constitutions have written out to what degree the right to an education is protected in that state. However, without federal oversight and mandates for education, even state constitutions can be violated. For instance, the California state constitution guarantees California children the right to an education, but as I've mentioned several times, California was last among the states in school reopening.

As Dr. Bienen points out, European countries kept schools open nearly the entire pandemic or instituted only short-term school closures to deal with specific COVID-19 waves. Indeed, European countries that kept schools open *do* specify the right to an education. Sweden's constitution spells out a right to an education, and Denmark's constitution even specifies a "child's right to psychical integrity and privacy" as well as protecting a child's right to an education.[123] Norway, which in 1739 became the first country to require compulsory primary education, also guarantees a right to higher education.[124] Article 14 of the European Union's charter states that the right to education includes free compulsory education, so even if an individual country's constitution does not spell out the right to an education, by joining the EU it must abide by the EU charter.[125] Australia, which lies somewhere between the United States and Europe in terms of school closures, also spells out a right to free education in its Human Rights Act.[126]

Dr. Bienen raises the point that the lack of focus on and attention to children's education in the United States may be in part due to our extreme protection of capitalism. Historically, the need for children to work during times of labor scarcity in the United States was in competition with their need to go to school. Codification of a commitment to children's rights—such as ratifying the 1989 UN Convention on the Rights of the Child (the United States is the only UN member not to have ratified this convention)—would go a long way. Finally, having federal protections for a right to an education, federal funding for public education, and a commitment to children's rights in the United States would do a lot to ensure that we balance the needs of children in our pandemic responses going forward.

RATIONAL DATA-DRIVEN POLICIES FOR MANAGING COVID AS AN ENDEMIC VIRUS IN SCHOOLS

As COVID becomes an endemic virus, it is important to plan rational, data-driven policies for schools in order to limit further harm to children. Though we will not be able to eradicate COVID, we can mitigate its harms and the harms of future pandemics while appropriately meeting children's needs. Vaccination and therapeutics will protect most vulnerable individuals from serious illness but, as with other respiratory pathogens, a small number of children and adults will be at risk. However, that number will be low enough to justify meeting other societal needs, similar to the way in which we accept the risks of influenza or driving. What we need to is to keep sick children out of school and emphasize mitigation strategies that are supported by robust evidence, such as vaccination and ventilation, not those that have less data showing their benefit, such as universal masking. Moving forward, each pandemic will need to be weighed differently in terms of the risks it poses (or not) to children, so this chapter is not a blanket prescription for all pandemics. But because the COVID-19 pandemic was remarkable in its relative sparing of young children, the inordinate burden that COVID restrictions in the United States placed on children was unjustified.

In February 2022, my colleague Dr. Daniel Johnson (professor of pediatrics at the University of Chicago Medicine, section chief for pediatric infectious diseases) and I proposed the following six steps as a road map for schools as COVID moved into the endemic stage:[127]

1. Focus efforts on vaccination for children and adults, particularly where vaccination rates are lowest due to issues of access to care, reduced vaccine confidence, and insufficient outreach.
2. Continue to upgrade school ventilation systems. Improved ventilation can significantly reduce the spread of the virus. This can be achieved through any combination of opening windows and doors, increasing ventilation rates in

mechanically ventilated buildings, using MERV-13 filters, and supplementing with portable air cleaners with HEPA filters.[128]

3. Stop asymptomatic testing and contact tracing.[129] Test-to-stay was the strategy whereby children who were exposed to COVID could test and stay in the classroom if negative. The largest study of the test-to-stay strategy showed no meaningful impact of asymptomatic testing and tracing on community transmission.[130] This supports the Children's Hospital of Philadelphia Policy Lab's recommendation to stop asymptomatic testing in schools in January 2022 (a recommendation not endorsed by the CDC until August 2022 and not fully implemented during times of CDC-defined high community transmission).

4. Return children to normal lunchtime socializing.[131] Free time is critical for children's social, emotional, and interpersonal development. It's time to nurture childhood friendships and strengthen the bonds of our school communities.

5. Retire mask mandates once hospitalization rates from COVID are low in the United States, since all non-pharmaceutical interventions were put into place to reduce transmission and protect hospitals. Encourage those who desire extra protection or whose medical team has recommended it to them to wear well-fitted N95 or similar masks.[132]

6. Scale up mental health services and social supports in schools. After two years of trauma, significant

resources—from in-school counselors to support
animals—will be needed to minimize the long-term
impact on students' mental and physical health.

The most recent National Assessment of Educational Progress
report shows that in 2022 scores in mathematics declined significantly among students in grades 4 and 8, with reading scores also
falling.[133] I have no doubt that this is a result of COVID-related
school closures. Given that vaccines were available for adults (teachers, staff, family members) in the United States since the spring of
2021 and that schools reopened so much earlier in Europe, this
report should trigger reflection along with educational recovery
efforts.

"Zero risk" is unobtainable, and an effort to drive case numbers to zero can have unintended negative effects, as evidenced by
the devastating consequences school closures have had on children's
health and safety. In the next pandemic, we can and must do better
by our children.

CHAPTER 6

The Need for Global Equity in COVID-19 Vaccines and Treatments

As of December 2022, only 25.1 percent of people in low-income countries had received at least one dose of a COVID-19 vaccine.[1] Even with high rates of natural infection and subsequent immunity during the omicron wave across the planet, receiving at least one dose of a COVID-19 vaccine, especially for older individuals, provides more durable and reliable hybrid immunity.[2]

During the delta surge, which was especially devastating in India, wealthy countries, including the United States, were debating whether COVID-19 vaccine patents should be waived, given the epic humanitarian crisis unfolding from the virus, the precedent for waiving patents in the context of public health emergencies, and the amazing real-world effectiveness of most COVID-19 vaccines against severe disease.[3] Heartbreaking scenes from India in the spring of 2021, from overflowing hospitals turning away dying patients to crematorium pyres burning all night, were actively playing out at the same time as debates on how fast wealthy countries with rapid vaccine rollouts would be getting back to normal life.[4]

Pharmaceutical companies producing COVID-19 vaccines and holding patents are reaping billions of dollars in profit from vaccines and booster shots in wealthy countries.[5] In October 2020, India and South Africa formally proposed to the World Trade Organization's Council for Trade-Related Aspects of Intellectual Property Rights (TRIPS) that intellectual property provisions for COVID-19 vaccines be temporarily waived so that India and other countries could mass-produce these vaccines for their populations.[6] On March 5, 2021 (as COVID-19 cases were just ramping up in India), CEOs of major pharmaceutical companies involved in COVID-19 vaccine production sent an open letter to President Biden urging him to reject this "unfortunate" proposal.[7]

To stay on the theme of how the lessons we've learned from HIV could have informed our response to COVID-19, this debate sounds all too familiar, as rigid adherence to patent laws directly led to millions of lives lost to HIV/AIDS in sub-Saharan Africa in the 1990s and 2000s, despite the development of highly effective antiretroviral therapies (ART) by 1996.[8] I recall directly witnessing plummeting AIDS-related mortality from the first half to the second half of my first year of internship at a hospital in San Francisco that year, a miracle afforded initially only to those with AIDS in wealthy countries.[9]

Pfizer made $41.9 billion in 2000, a year when HIV activists and doctors were aghast that the company's patented antifungal fluconazole (which could be made for pennies) was priced so high that it remained unaffordable for countries in sub-Saharan Africa.[10] Fluconazole was the only treatment for cryptococcal meningitis, an AIDS-related opportunistic infection with a high mortality rate if untreated.[11] AIDS patients in Africa needlessly died of cryptococcal meningitis due to lack of access to a patented drug until South Africa openly defied patent laws.[12] Meanwhile, in 2000, the pharmaceutical industry spent $167 million on lobbying during the US election campaign, more than was spent by any other industry.[13] Lifesaving ART medications were not available for most poor countries for years and years after they were approved in the United States in 1996. In 2001, Kofi Annan, the UN secretary general, said, "Some may think that because better medicines have been found, the AIDS emergency is over. Alas, no. For most people living with HIV/AIDS today, the $10,000 to $60,000 annual price tag of an anti-retroviral regime belongs, quite simply, in another galaxy."[14]

The debate about waiving patents raged on during the early 2000s, as millions continued to die of AIDS in poor countries.[15] The WTO's TRIPS agreement, ratified in 1995, had allowed for patent waivers and domestic production off-patent in the setting of medical emergencies, but with patent laws intact, ART regimens remained out of reach for the majority of poor patients in sub-Saharan Africa throughout this period.[16] In early 2001, an Indian pharmaceutical company named Cipla (which focused on the production of generic medicines) decided to offer a triple-combination ART regimen at $350 per patient per year—less than a dollar a day.[17] US- and Europe-based pharmaceutical companies making ART medications opposed this offer from India to inexpensively manufacture ART for poor regions across the world, so the Treatment Action Campaign (TAC), a long-standing HIV advocacy organization in South Africa, took the dispute to the world stage by distributing the inexpensive Cipla-made ART regimen without approval. Large pharmaceutical companies countered by launching a lawsuit against the South African government and TAC. However, this lawsuit "hammered the message home that many of the multinational drug companies were abusing their market monopoly in the face of a catastrophic human disaster" and, under increasing international pressure, the lawsuit was dropped.[18] To this day, only

76 percent of adults and 52 percent of children among the 38.4 million people living with HIV worldwide have access to lifesaving ART, with 650,000 deaths from AIDS recorded in 2021.[19] My options for prescribing ART regimens for patients living with HIV in wealthy countries are much more diverse and plentiful than options for those in resource-limited settings, due to strict patent laws. On the other hand, I am grateful for the advocacy from the international community that took place in the early 2000s to reach this place of expanded ART access worldwide in 2022.

Unlike with HIV, for which the decision to waive patent laws on some ART regimens took years of activist pressure, the decision on waiving patents for COVID-19 vaccines needed to be made more quickly, as COVID-19 was a global public health emergency. When the delta variant hit India, only 9.2 percent of Indians had received their first dose of COVID-19 vaccine.[20] Immediate waiving of pharmaceutical company patents in the face of this wide-scale human tragedy, so that vaccine production could be increased for and by India, would have been an obvious next step. India supplied ART to the world in the 2000s; it was our duty to help India when COVID-19 hit. As the United Nations secretary general said in February 2021, "Vaccine equity is the biggest moral test before the global community" at this time.[21] Although COVID-19 vaccines saved 20 million lives during the first year of their rollout, millions more lives would have been saved in low- and middle-income countries if we had had greater global vaccine equity after the vaccine was developed. We therefore failed the moral test highlighted by the UN.[22]

Now that oral antiviral treatments have been approved for COVID-19, we also need to expand access for low-income countries to these medications for those who are at risk of severe breakthrough infections (Chapter 3). The pharmaceutical companies that invented Paxlovid and molnupiravir both signed on to the Medicines Patent Pool in late 2021, which will immediately allow generic manufacturers to produce these lifesaving medications and expand access to them in low- and middle-income countries.[23]

Beyond questions of waiving patents, the United States could foster the spread of lifesaving vaccines by encouraging public-private partnerships through voluntary licensing agreements to increase manufacturing capacity.[24] The United States could also support increased production of particular materials, such as the lipid particles used to encase the mRNA in the mRNA vaccines, to accelerate global manufacturing.

On March 30, 2022, the WHO issued a road map for moving on from the emergency phase of the pandemic.[25] It put forth three different possible scenarios in terms of the need for ongoing booster vaccines: (1) a baseline scenario (current omicron era), in which vulnerable populations such as immunocompromised and older individuals would need to be boosted every winter; (2) a best-case scenario (if a less virulent variant emerges), in which most people will not need a booster; and (3) a worst-case scenario (if a more virulent variant emerges), in which everyone who is eligible will need a booster vaccination.

If we look in more detail at some elements of the first, baseline scenario, it can help us pinpoint who is likely to need boosters and when. One research study has shown that a single booster has a very strong protective effect against severe disease from the BA1 and BA2 strains of the omicron variant, with boosted individuals continuing to demonstrate the powerful cellular immunity (from T and B cells) triggered by the vaccines.[26] Another research study shows that a single booster with an mRNA vaccine provides additional protection for at least six months, so we can estimate six months as the minimum interval between boosters.[27] A third study shows that giving boosters too early after an infection (within sixty days) actually makes the immune response to the booster less effective.[28] A fourth study identified people sixty-five and older as those still at risk of severe breakthrough infection during omicron and concluded that they should be prescribed Paxlovid if they get infected, in order to prevent hospitalization.[29] Therefore, older people and immunocompromised people will benefit from boosters during times of high viral circulation, which is likely to be in the winter, as COVID-19 settles into a pattern more common with other respiratory pathogens, such as colds and flu. In these individuals, a booster provides an immediate initial surge of antibodies, which is helpful because B cells exposed to a pathogen typically take two to four days to make neutralizing antibodies, and in people who are more susceptible to severe disease this may be too long to wait.[30]

At some point, the United States will also need to clarify the goals of our booster strategy.[31] If the aim is to prevent severe disease (as has been articulated by other countries and endorsed by the WHO), we likely will only be giving regular boosters to older and immunocompromised individuals.[32]

Given that SARS-CoV-2 is a non-eradicable virus, keeping COVID-19 in the endemic phase will require continued investment in vaccines and therapeutics and a commitment to the global community for equitable access. On April 5, 2022, the International Monetary Fund estimated that $10 billion annually will be needed to combat COVID-19 worldwide.[33] This commitment to fight COVID-19—and other pandemics, as well as to strengthen health systems worldwide—is critical.

CHAPTER 7

A Post-Pandemic Playbook

n November 2021, I coauthored with other public health experts a peer-reviewed piece titled "Revisiting COVID-19 Policies: 10 Evidence-Based Recommendations for Where to Go from Here," which was published in *BMC Public Health*.[1] Although our suggestions there are specific to the COVID-19 pandemic, many lessons from this pandemic can be applied as a potential playbook for future pandemics.

I recommend the following strategies for future pandemics, to accomplish the dual goal of minimizing suffering and death from the pathogen and taking the holistic needs of society into account using principles of harm reduction. A long history of work in HIV medicine and research has taught me and others how to harness biomedical tools for the pathogen while taking the larger needs of individuals and societies into account. With biomedical interventions for pathogens, we can both save the lives of those infected and minimize damage to other aspects of public health, including public trust.

ACCELERATE VACCINATION

Pandemic phases or outbreaks of infectious diseases usually come to an end through population immunity, unless there is not an effective vaccine or immune response to the pathogen. In the case of

COVID-19, we have both developed effective vaccines and come to understand how immunity to the virus develops, either through vaccination or through natural infection. By contrast, for HIV there has so far been no effective vaccine developed and no way to date to elicit an effective immune response to clear the virus. That's largely because of the nature of the virus. Unlike the coronavirus SARS-CoV-2, HIV is a retrovirus—it starts out as an RNA virus, but once inside a human host, its genetic material is converted to DNA. This DNA inserts itself into the human host chromosome, turning HIV into a chronic infection. Human immunity is ineffective in ousting this indwelling virus, and an HIV vaccine so far has been elusive (although new mRNA HIV vaccine trials are underway and promising). HIV—although it can be controlled with treatments and preventatives—is nowhere near coming to an end.

Steps for Pandemic Management (figure designed by Karina Escandón for the manuscript "Revisiting COVID-19 Policies: 10 Evidence-Based Recommendations for Where to Go from Here," *BMC Public Health*, 2021)

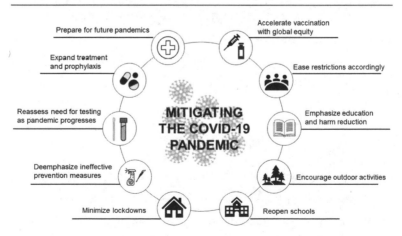

For pathogens like SARS-CoV-2, to which the human body can mount an effective immune response, vaccination is a much safer way to acquire immunity than enduring the natural infection. However, natural immunity has controlled disease in prior infectious disease pandemics. As we've seen, the 1918 influenza pandemic was by far the deadliest respiratory virus pandemic recorded in recent human history, but the fatal consequences of this highly transmissible virus slowed only after enough of the population had acquired immunity, since the first vaccine for influenza was not developed until 1942.[2] And measles is a highly transmissible respiratory virus that prior to the development of a vaccine in 1963 caused deaths each year among the nonimmune.[3] Similarly, infection with smallpox (and many other pathogens for which we have developed vaccines) also led to natural immunity, but often with concomitant severe disease and death.[4]

The progress in developing and approving COVID-19 vaccines within a year of the time the WHO declared the virus a pandemic is unprecedented. As Dr. Barney Graham, coinventor of the COVID mRNA vaccine, wrote in 2018, "Despite the impending threat of pandemic disease from emerging viruses, the ability and technological tools are available to achieve a substantial level of advanced preparation before the next major event, and if a systematic effort can be sustained, effective interventions for the majority of future pathogens can be developed."[5] The mRNA vaccine technology is not new, but COVID-19 represented the first time this technology came into wide-scale use.[6] For all future pandemics, vaccines will be our first line of defense, and we now have the tools to develop and deploy them quickly. Scientists should patiently explain the known safety of the mRNA vaccine technology, along with other vaccine platforms, and insist on global vaccine equity to combat a pandemic.[7] Although misinformation regarding COVID-19 vaccines hampered their uptake in the United States, acknowledging that different types of vaccines have different adverse effects and providing the option for personalized medicine by providing a variety of vaccine options will increase trust.

Maximizing global vaccine production and equitable distribution must be the highest priority, and we should seek out innovative mechanisms of financing and licensing production that will make this possible. The wealthier countries should largely pay for this ongoing effort as a humanitarian imperative as well as from enlightened self-interest. Because at the start of any vaccine response availability of the vaccine is likely to be limited, strategies should include prioritizing vulnerable populations and healthcare workers and delaying doses for those with previous infection until those without prior immunity are vaccinated. If a vaccine requires two doses, delaying the second dose for longer than the interval used in clinical trials will increase overall public health benefit by maximizing coverage with first doses more quickly and also lead to a better immune response.

In sum, in future pandemics we should generally advocate for approaches that offer the most people some protection as quickly as possible. High-income countries should be exhorted to deploy any soon-to-expire doses overseas and to join the WHO's COVID-19 Technology Access Pool, which would allow other countries to produce patented vaccines, thereby expanding their availability in low- and middle-income countries. International governance of vaccine distribution is essential in order to address vaccine inequity and to maximize positive outcomes globally.

EASE RESTRICTIONS ON POPULATIONS

As vaccines are deployed, restrictions on the population should be quickly eased.[8] We have seen excess mortality from restrictions imposed during COVID-19, including an increase in alcohol use, substance use, overdose deaths, gun violence, and the consequences of shutting down medical care for other chronic medical conditions. Moreover, countries that quickly pivoted to normalcy after vaccine deployment fared better in terms of vaccine uptake and trust in public health. Vaccine uptake in the United States was not as high as in other high-income countries, leading to avoidable deaths here.[9]

As early as February 2021, I said that to promote vaccine uptake we should message optimism about the vaccines, specifically how they could help us get back to normal life.[10] Acknowledging people's strong desire for normalcy could have been a major motivator of vaccine uptake in our country. I think the White House's confusing messaging, suggesting a need to mask after vaccination and that life does not go back to normal even after getting vaccinated, negatively affected vaccine uptake. A one-size-fits-all approach in terms of booster recommendations by the White House (e.g., saying *everyone* needed a booster in the winter of 2022 instead of only older immunocompromised individuals) also likely reduced trust. Other countries, like Denmark and Switzerland, messaged more optimism about the vaccines and went back to normal life after high rates of vaccination, unlike the United States.

Moreover, although I was an early supporter of masks, mask mandates didn't seem to make much of a difference in the United States, as covered in Chapter 3.[11] Acknowledging that the randomized controlled clinical trials data on population masking during the COVID-19 pandemic did not provide a strong premise for mask mandates (versus mask recommendations) will help increase trust in public health.

EMPHASIZE EDUCATION AND HARM REDUCTION APPROACHES OVER COERCIVE AND PUNITIVE MEASURES

We have covered this at length in other chapters, but abstinence-only approaches have not worked for AIDS or teen pregnancy prevention, and similarly absolutist approaches have not worked well for preventing SARS-CoV-2, either.[12] Instead, prevention measures should be founded on the provision of accurate information that is sensitively communicated and should be informed by harm reduction approaches that are more effective and sustainable in the longer term.[13] As we've seen, harm reduction involves giving people the information and tools they need to assess and mitigate risk, while acknowledging the real-world conditions that may lead some persons to take calculated risks.

Before the vaccines were rolled out, one example of a successful COVID-19 mitigation campaign that didn't involve shutting everything down completely was the "Three Cs" approach in Japan, which advised people to avoid (1) closed spaces with poor ventilation, (2) crowded places with many people nearby, and (3) close-contact settings.[14] Educating the public about effective precautions, including vaccination, and motivating people to adopt those precautions are more effective than coercive or punitive measures (e.g., shaming, fines, imprisonment, and even police violence) and will help alleviate pandemic response fatigue.[15] Trusting that populations will want to stay safe is more effective than authoritarian measures such as those imposed in China for so long. Accordingly, any restrictions and mandates, including vaccination passports or mandates, should focus on high-risk situations and consider the relevant scientific and ethical questions.[16]

Most importantly, pandemic control measures should be formulated and reassessed based on the latest information, levels of ongoing threat, and resource availability.

ENCOURAGE OUTDOOR ACTIVITIES FOR RESPIRATORY PATHOGEN CONTROL

Current evidence on the transmission dynamics of SARS-CoV-2 must inform policy recommendations for mitigation strategies and restrictions.[17] Unfortunately, at many points during the pandemic lower-risk activities, especially those conducted in outdoor environments (e.g., parks, beaches, hiking trails, playgrounds), were discouraged or even prohibited.[18] The risk of SARS-CoV-2 transmission outdoors is vastly lower than it is indoors, with most studies finding the proportion of new cases attributable to outdoor exposure to be less than 1 percent.[19] Policies should reflect this enormous difference in risk, including allowing access to outdoor spaces even during periods of severe restrictions and reserving mask mandates for indoor situations, as recommended by the WHO.[20] Strongly encouraging outdoor activities and including nuance in public health recommendations are more consistent with harm-reduction-based approaches.[21]

When weather or other factors preclude holding activities outdoors, windows should be kept open whenever possible, including in shared vehicles, and ventilation (at least four air exchanges per hour) should be ensured to reduce the risk of transmission.[22]

REOPEN SCHOOLS AS SOON AS FEASIBLE

Given the essential nature of school for children's development and well-being (see Chapter 5), schools should be reopened as soon as possible when confronting a pandemic. The fact that children were so much less at risk of severe disease with SARS-CoV-2 should have guided policies on school openings in this particular pandemic. The response in future pandemics will depend on the severity of the infection in children, although in other infectious disease pandemics throughout history, school closures have generally been kept to a minimum. Performing good studies on the necessity of different mitigation procedures in schools and comparing outcomes across countries (including the Scandinavian countries, which generally had the shortest duration of closed schools and the fewest restrictions on children) will be important in future pandemics.

MINIMIZE LOCKDOWNS

The cumulative evidence suggests that sledgehammer-like lockdown approaches, such as the closing of all nonessential workplaces and schools, should be avoided in favor of more effective, carefully targeted scalpel-like public health strategies.[23] Indiscriminate lockdowns have had far-reaching unintended consequences, disproportionately affecting socioeconomically disadvantaged and vulnerable populations. Other consequences include alarming increases in mental health problems (depression, anxiety, and social isolation), drug overdoses, domestic violence, child abuse, weight gain, and discontinuation of clinical services and prevention programs.[24]

Tailored, context-sensitive interventions involving fewer economic, societal, and quality-of-life costs than lockdowns are likely to be more effective and minimize harm. Non-pharmaceutical interventions (NPIs) such as physical distancing, improved ventilation, and effective indoor mask wearing are also more sustainable than broad stay-at-home orders.[25] When lockdowns, isolation, or quarantine measures are mandated, economic hardship should be considered and paid sick/quarantine leaves and other types of support must be provided to affected workers, especially those who are the most economically vulnerable.[26]

In the winter of 2022, another effect of lockdowns, NPIs, and school closures emerged: the "immunity debt," the concept that a greater proportion of the population is more susceptible to disease after a long period of reduced exposure. This led to higher rates and more severe disease with respiratory syncytial virus (RSV) and influenza among children and older adults.[27]

DEEMPHASIZE INEFFECTIVE MEASURES
AS SOON AS POSSIBLE

Given the respiratory transmission route of SARS-CoV-2, physical distancing, one-way masking with fit and filtered masks (N95, KN95, FFP2, and KF94 masks), and improved ventilation are the most effective NPIs.[28] On the other hand, the evidence is consistent that transmission via a contaminated surface is not a significant driver of SARS-CoV-2 spread, as the CDC has acknowledged.[29] Many of the disinfection rituals we adopted during the pandemic, including the ubiquitous usage of alcohol-based hand sanitizers and the excessive use of strong cleaning products, are unnecessary to prevent the spread of COVID; in fact, misuse of such products, such as washing food with bleach, applying household cleaners or disinfectants to bare skin, mixing bleach solutions with vinegar or ammonia, and intentionally or accidentally inhaling or ingesting such products, has resulted in toxic reactions, occasionally leading to hospitalization and even death.[30] Beyond being ineffective and occasionally dangerous, excessive cleaning rituals divert important resources, time, attention, and energy from more useful forms of prevention.[31] There are also growing concerns about the potential longer-term impacts of excessive use of antimicrobial substances on antimicrobial resistance rates in the future.[32] Public health authorities (and the media) must do a much better job of educating the public how the coronavirus is—and is not—typically transmitted.[33] For example, fleeting encounters and surfaces pose extremely minimal risk, even with more transmissible variants.

Another pervasive practice, temperature screening—especially when using handheld noncontact infrared thermometers—is often inaccurate due to environmental factors (e.g., distance between subject and sensor, ambient temperature, humidity), operator-dependent performance, and device variability.[34] Furthermore, fever is a poor differentiator of the presence or absence of SARS-CoV-2 infection (and the use of antipyretic drugs may mask fever). A systematic review of studies regarding exit and entry screening practices (e.g., symptom questionnaires, body temperature measurement) during previous epidemics of influenza A (H1N1), Ebola, and severe acute respiratory syndrome (SARS) found that these practices were of extremely low or no utility in differentiating infected people from uninfected people.[35] For COVID-19, similar findings have been reported, with only a very small proportion of SARS-CoV-2 infections detected with such screening practices.[36] Again, such measures divert resources and attention away from much more effective strategies to control infection.

Furthermore, travel-related restrictions have clearly had a considerable impact on global trade and economies as well as on other systems, including those for international humanitarian responses.[37] Other negative consequences include generating a false sense of security, discouraging travelers from being truthful when questioned by authorities, and potentially disincentivizing open disclosure by countries during future outbreaks.[38] Although a few countries (e.g., New Zealand, Australia, Taiwan, China), mainly island nations, have attempted to eliminate SARS-CoV-2 through use of robust quarantine and contact tracing measures, it makes little sense, from either an epidemiological or a human rights perspective, to shut international land borders or require a negative PCR test result for entry into countries where SARS-CoV-2 is already circulating widely.[39] Similarly, the routine use of quarantine upon arrival and various other entrance screening procedures are also largely ineffective. Such border controls are akin to confiscating matches after the forest is already ablaze.[40] Experience, including lessons learned during this pandemic, suggests that imposition of travel restrictions also generally fails to prevent the spread of new genetic variants, as their discovery typically lags well behind their emergence, and local detection often depends more on which locations are conducting routine genomic surveillance than on where the new variants actually originate.[41]

REASSESS TESTING PRACTICES AND POLICIES

Experience suggests that choice of diagnostic technologies should be determined by the intended use, whether to detect infection in individuals with suspected clinical symptoms or to identify potentially infectious individuals in order to inform isolation recommendations and conduct contact tracing. PCR-based assays were the preferred method for much too long in the pandemic, despite being too sensitive.[42] Rapid antigen tests, which are both cheaper and faster, can lead to false negatives, especially in presymptomatic carriers and when conducted without adequate quality control procedures, and to false positives, when cases in the surrounding community are low. However, if performed by trained technicians in appropriate populations, they may be sufficiently sensitive and specific for detecting potential infectiousness, thus suggesting that antigen tests should be the preferred method for public health screening.[43] Moreover, further investigation is needed regarding the extent to which positive SARS-CoV-2 PCR or antigen results do not always reflect actual infectiousness or viral viability, particularly among populations of vaccinated or asymptomatic individuals.[44] Finally, given that vaccination reduces symptomatic and asymptomatic SARS-CoV-2 infections and that vaccinated individuals are likely to be less infectious if infected, testing and quarantine of vaccinated (or previously infected) persons following exposure to someone with suspected or confirmed COVID-19 should in general only be needed if COVID-19 symptoms develop.[45]

As we increasingly recognize that SARS-CoV-2 is gradually becoming an endemic virus, it is vital to deemphasize identification of new cases (through mass asymptomatic testing) as the way we measure the effectiveness of mitigation measures; rather, we should assess mortality and hospitalization rates.[46] This is especially relevant considering that the vaccines reduce severe and fatal outcomes from COVID-19 but do not prevent all infections.

EXPAND ACCESS TO OUTPATIENT
THERAPIES AND PROPHYLACTICS

As with vaccines, the pandemic has presented challenges in identifying effective therapeutics on a greatly accelerated timeline. Although vaccination remains the priority, some vaccinated individuals will still contract SARS-CoV-2, and some persons will remain unvaccinated. Approved outpatient therapies for COVID-19 are mainly oral antivirals, and these should be provided worldwide. As evidence on treatment options evolves, policymakers should prioritize quick access to effective outpatient therapies—such as molnupiravir and Paxlovid—in patients with risk factors for severe disease. The study of previously identified safe medications might be a novel and efficient way to quickly identify new therapies.[47] New oral protease inhibitors are being developed and tested. In addition, more research is urgently needed regarding the prevalence, diagnosis, prognosis, and treatment options for PASC (long COVID).

PREVENT AND PREPARE FOR FUTURE PANDEMICS

COVID-19 is the second major respiratory viral pandemic in a century and the third coronavirus that has caused severe disease within two decades. More pandemics are likely in the coming years, from new coronaviruses and/or from other pathogens. We clearly must do everything possible to prevent and be better prepared for future pandemics and other public health emergencies, and we must learn and apply lessons from our recent experience with COVID-19.[48]

Regarding prevention, policymakers must take prudent actions immediately to reduce the likelihood of future pandemics, including addressing the environmental destruction that brings different nonhuman species into closer contact with humans, restricting the trafficking of exotic animals, and strengthening biosecurity in laboratories that work with potential human pathogens.

In preparation for the next pandemics, international organizations should come up with detailed plans that are widely vetted and agreed upon. Lockdowns and quarantines, when (and only if) necessary, need to be designed with attention to equity and must include protection, prioritization, and compensation for those most vulnerable, including the elderly, the poor, and workers in front-line and informal jobs.[49] Effective mechanisms must also be established to address equity in access to treatments and vaccines, prioritizing those at highest risk. We certainly must avoid another situation in which public health authorities and politicians are left to fly blind and then try to clean up the damage later. It would be a grave error to respond to a new pandemic without applying lessons from the current one.

Acknowledgments

I would like to acknowledge Linh Pham, medical and graduate student (M.D./Ph.D.) at the University of Texas, San Antonio, who researched a lot of the papers and formulated the structure of Chapter 5. Pranay Narang, undergraduate student at Nova Southeastern University and premedical student, significantly contributed to this book by compiling and organizing references. Nishan Sohoni, undergraduate student at the University of Southern California and premedical student, additionally worked on Chapter 5 and contributed to the learning loss section in particular. Joseph Watabe, my amazing administrative assistant, contributed to reference compilation and simply makes my life possible every day. I would like to also thank my agent at Watermark Agency, Mark Tauber, who was patient with my initial reluctance to compile these thoughts (which is harder to do than to compose tweets!) but saw me through to the end. And, finally, I would like to thank my sons, Ishaan and Vedant, who watched me spend way too much time on this after their father passed and were very happy when I sent it off! And thanks to my parents, brother, sister, father-in-law, mother-in-law, and friends, who all supported me through the death of my husband and this COVID-related work. I hope this contributes to the knowledge base on COVID and allows us to think differently about managing the next pandemic in light of the lessons from HIV. Thank you all so much!

Notes

INTRODUCTION

1. CDC, "Pneumocystis Pneumonia—Los Angeles," *Morbidity and Mortality Weekly Report,* June 5, 1981, https://www.cdc.gov/mmwr/preview/mmwrhtml/june_5.htm; CDC, "Kaposi's Sarcoma and Pneumocystis Pneumonia Among Homosexual Men—New York City and California," *Morbidity and Mortality Weekly Report,* July 4, 1981; 30: 305–308.
2. Gandhi M, "Overcaution Carries Its Own Danger to Children," *The Atlantic,* February 27, 2021, https://www.theatlantic.com/ideas/archive/2021/02/vaccines-are-banishing-any-debate-about-reopening-schools/618155/; Henderson TO, Gandhi M, Hoeg TB, Johnson D, "CDC Misinterpreted Our Research on Opening Schools. It Should Loosen the Rules Now," *USA Today,* March 9, 2021, https://www.usatoday.com/story/opinion/2021/03/09/cdc-school-opening-COVID-rules-guidance-column/4628552001/; Hoeg TB, Henderson T, Johnson D, Gandhi M, "Our Next National Priority Should Be to Reopen All America's Schools for Full Time In-Person Learning," *The Hill,* March 20, 2021, https://thehill.com/opinion/healthcare/544142-our-next-national-priority-should-be-to-reopen-all-americas-schools-for/; Bienen L, Happel E, Gandhi M, "Real-World Data, Not Predictions, Should Drive Decisions on COVID-19 and School Opening," *Stat,* April 23, 2021, https://www.statnews.com/2021/04/23/use-real-world-data-not-predictions-inform-school-opening-decisions/; Noble J, Gandhi M, "Is It Safe to Fully Reopen California Schools? It's Not Unsafe Not To, Says UCSF's Jeanne Noble and Monica Gandhi," *San Francisco Chronicle,* June 4, 2021, https://www.sfchronicle.com/opinion/openforum/article/Is-it-safe-to-fully-reopen-California-schools-16224689.php; Hoeg TB,

Gandhi M, Johnson D, "We Must Fully Reopen Schools This Fall. Here's How," *New York Times,* June 8, 2021, https://www.nytimes.com/2021/06/08/opinion/blueprint-reopening-schools.html; Gandhi M, Noble J, "The Pandemic's Toll on Teen Mental Health," *Wall Street Journal,* June 10, 2021, https://www.wsj.com/articles/the-pandemics-toll-on-teen-mental-health-11623344542; Vergales J, Gandhi M, "School Quarantines Keep Too Many Kids at Home—with Barely Any Effect on COVID," *Washington Post,* October 5, 2021, https://www.washingtonpost.com/outlook/2021/10/05/quarantine-COVID-schools-modified-test/; Gandhi M, Johnson D, "A Roadmap to COVID-19 Endemicity in Schools," Smerconish, February 5, 2022, https://www.smerconish.com/exclusive-content/a-roadmap-to-COVID-19-endemicity-in-schools/.

3. Gandhi M, "We Won't Eradicate COVID-19. The Pandemic Will Still End," *Washington Post,* September 21, 2020, https://www.washingtonpost.com/outlook/2021/09/21/COVID-pandemic-end/.

4. Strassburg MA, "The Global Eradication of Smallpox," *American Journal of Infection Control* 10, no. 2 (May 1982): 53–59, https://doi.org/10.1016/0196-6553(82)90003-7.

5. Crist C, "COVID-19 Found in 29 Types of Animals, Scientists Say," WebMD, March 7, 2022, https://www.webmd.com/lung/news/20220307/COVID-found-in-29-types-of-animals; Willgert K, Didelot X, Surendran-Nair M, et al., "Transmission History of SARS-CoV-2 in Humans and White-Tailed Deer," *Scientific Reports* 12: 12094, https://doi.org/10.1038/s41598-022-16071-z.

6. Gandhi, "We Won't Eradicate COVID-19."

7. Thompson D, "School Closures Were a Failed Policy," *The Atlantic,* October 2022, https://www.theatlantic.com/newsletters/archive/2022/10/pandemic-school-closures-americas-learning-loss/671868/.

8. Tulchinsky TH, "John Snow, Cholera, the Broad Street Pump; Waterborne Diseases Then and Now," *Case Studies in Public Health* 2018: 77–99, https://doi.org/10.1016/b978-0-12-804571-8.00017-2.

9. Ambrus A, Field E, Gonzalez R, "Loss in the Time of Cholera: Long-Run Impact of a Disease Epidemic on the Urban Landscape," *American Economic Review* 110, no. 2 (2020): 475–525, https://doi.org/10.1257/aer.20190759; Gandhi M, Prasad V, Baral S, "What Does Public Health Really Mean? Lessons from COVID-19," *British Medical Journal* blog, July 26, 2021, https://blogs.bmj.com/bmj/2021/07/26/what-does-public-health-really-mean-lessons-from-COVID-19/.

10. United Nations, Sustainable Development Goals, "SDG Moment | 19 September 2022," https://www.un.org/sustainabledevelopment/sdg -moment/.

11. UNICEF, "Impacts on Child Poverty: Social Policy Analysis to Inform the COVID-19 Response," accessed November 1, 2022, https://www .unicef.org/social-policy/child-poverty/COVID-19-socioeconomic -impacts; UNICEF, "Impact of COVID-19 on Multidimensional Child Poverty," September 2020, https://data.unicef.org/resources /impact-of-COVID-19-on-multidimensional-child-poverty/.

12. Galvani AP, Parpia AS, Pandey A, Zimmer C, Kahn JG, Fitzpatrick MC, "The Imperative for Universal Healthcare to Curtail the COVID-19 Outbreak in the USA," *eClinicalMedicine* 23 (2020): 100380, https:// www.thelancet.com/journals/eclinm/article/PIIS2589-5370(20)30124-3 /fulltext.

13. Gandhi M, "The Most Important Thing Rich Countries Can Do to Help India Fight COVID-19," *Time,* May 4, 2021, https://time .com/6046096/india-COVID-19-vaccine-patents/; Gandhi M, Wilkes M, "A Year with COVID Vaccines and We're Not Even Close to Ending Global Pandemic," *San Francisco Chronicle,* December 15, 2021, https://www.sfchronicle.com/opinion/openforum/article /Monica-Gandhi-and-Michael-Wilkes-A-year-with-16699634 .php; Gandhi M, "Four Ways HIV Activists Saved Lives During COVID," *Newsweek,* April 12, 2021, https://www.newsweek.com /four-ways-hiv-activists-saved-lives-during-COVID-opinion-1582504.

14. "The End of the COVID-19 Pandemic Is in Sight: WHO," UN News, September 14, 2022, https://news.un.org/en/story/2022/09/1126621.

15. Sacerdote BI, Sehgal R, Cook M, "Why Is All COVID-19 News Bad News?," Working Paper No. 28110, National Bureau of Economic Research, 2020, https://www.nber.org/papers/w28110; Xiong J, Lipsitz O, Nasri F, Lui LMW, Gill H, Phan L, Chen-Li D, et al., "Impact of COVID-19 Pandemic on Mental Health in the General Population: A Systematic Review," *Journal of Affective Disorders* 277 (2020): 55–64, https://doi.org/10.1016/j.jad.2020.08.001.

16. "The Week in Review: September 19–23," *Psychiatric Times,* September 24, 2022, https://www.psychiatrictimes.com/view/the-week-in-review -september-19-23.

17. Carlson CJ, Albery GF, Merow C, Trisos CH, Zipfel CM, Eskew EA, Olival KJ, Ross N, Bansal S, "Climate Change Increases Cross-Species Viral Transmission Risk," *Nature* 607, no. 7919 (2022): 555–562, https://

doi.org/10.1038/s41586-022-04788-w; Latkin CA, Dayton L, Strickland JC, Colon B, Rimal R, Boodram B, "An Assessment of the Rapid Decline of Trust in US Sources of Public Information About COVID-19," *Journal of Health Communication* 25, no. 10 (2020): 764–773, https://doi.org /10.1080/10810730.2020.1865487; WHO and UNICEF, "COVID-19 Pandemic Fuels Largest Continued Backslide in Vaccinations in Three Decades," July 15, 2022, https://www.who.int/news/item/15 -07-2022-COVID-19-pandemic-fuels-largest-continued-backslide-in -vaccinations-in-three-decades.

18. Oldekop JA, Horner R, Hulme D, Adhikari R, Agarwal B, Alford M, Bakewell O, et al., "COVID-19 and the Case for Global Development," *World Development* 134 (2020): 105044, https://doi.org/10.1016 /j.worlddev.2020.105044.

CHAPTER 1: HIV AS PROPHET AND TEACHER FOR COVID-19

1. Gandhi M, "Four Ways HIV Activists Saved Lives During COVID," *Newsweek,* April 12, 2021, https://www.newsweek.com /four-ways-hiv-activists-saved-lives-during-COVID-opinion-1582504.

2. Boyd GM, "Reagan Urges Abstinence for Young to Avoid AIDS," *New York Times,* April 2, 1987, https://www.nytimes.com/1987/04/02/us /reagan-urges-abstinence-for-young-to-avoid-aids.html.

3. Lewis T, "How the U.S. Pandemic Response Went Wrong—and What Went Right—During a Year of COVID," *Scientific American,* March 2021, https://www.scientificamerican.com/article/how-the-u-s -pandemic-response-went-wrong-and-what-went-right-during-a-year -of-COVID/.

4. Sacerdote BI, Sehgal R, Cook M, "Why Is All COVID-19 News Bad News?," Working Paper No. 28110, National Bureau of Economic Research, November 2020, https://www.nber.org/papers/w28110.

5. Leonhardt D, "Bad News Bias," *New York Times,* March 24, 2021, https://www.nytimes.com/2021/03/24/briefing/boulder-shooting -george-segal-astrazeneca.html.

6. Kupferschmidt K, "Will the Pandemic Fade into an Ordinary Disease Like the Flu? The World Is Watching Denmark for Clues," *Science,* September 30, 2021, https://www.science.org/content/article/will -pandemic-fade-ordinary-disease-flu-world-watching-denmark-clues; Kingsley P, "In Denmark, the Rarest of Sights: Classrooms Full of

Students," *New York Times,* April 17, 2020, https://www.nytimes
.com/2020/04/17/world/europe/denmark-schools-coronavirus
.html.

7. Harper CA, Satchell D, Fido D, et al., "Functional Fear Predicts Public
Health Compliance in the COVID-19 Pandemic," *International Journal
of Mental Health and Addiction* 19, no. 5 (2021): 1875–1888, https://
link.springer.com/article/10.1007/s11469-020-00281-5.

8. Jemmott JB, Jemmott LS, Fong GT, "Abstinence and Safer Sex HIV
Risk-Reduction Interventions for African American Adolescents:
A Randomized Controlled Trial," *Journal of the American Medical
Association* 279, no. 19 (1998): 1529–1536, https://jamanetwork.com
/journals/jama/fullarticle/187546.

9. Frampton B, "Clickbait: The Changing Face of Online Journalism,"
BBC News, September 14, 2015, https://www.bbc.com/news/uk-wales
-34213693.

10. Mueller B, "Nearly Half of COVID Patients Haven't Fully Recovered
Months Later, Study Finds," *New York Times,* October 12, 2022, www
.nytimes.com/2022/10/12/health/long-COVID.html.

11. *"Pneumocystis* Pneumonia—Los Angeles," *Morbidity and Mortality
Weekly Report,* June 5, 1981, https://www.cdc.gov/mmwr/preview/mmw
rhtml/june_5.htm.

12. Gallo RC, Montagnier L, "The Discovery of HIV as the Cause of AIDS,"
New England Journal of Medicine 349, no. 24 (2003): 2283–2285, https://
www.nejm.org/doi/full/10.1056/nejmp038194.

13. Abramson M, "How AIDS Remained an Unspoken—but Deadly—
Epidemic for Years," History.com, June 1, 2020, https://www.history
.com/news/aids-epidemic-ronald-reagan.

14. Hubley D, "Did Closing New York City Bathhouses in the 1980s Strip
Dignity from Gay Men?," Bates News, March 16, 2018, https://www
.bates.edu/news/2018/03/16/did-the-1980s-closure-of-nycs-bathhouses
-strip-dignity-from-gay-men/; Pulerwitz J, "How Stigma Subverts Public
Health," *Nature,* November 19, 2019, https://www.nature.com/articles
/d41586-019-03531-2.

15. Boyd GM, "Reagan Urges Abstinence for Young to Avoid AIDS," *New
York Times,* April 2, 1987, https://www.nytimes.com/1987/04/02/us
/reagan-urges-abstinence-for-young-to-avoid-aids.html; Gandhi M,
"Monkeypox and COVID: Public Health Has to Increase Trust,"
Medscape, June 28, 2022, https://www.medscape.com/viewarticle
/976081; Pulerwitz J, "How Stigma Subverts Public Health," *Nature,*

November 19, 2019, https://www.nature.com/articles/d41586-019
-03531-2.

16. Chan CA et al., "Harm Reduction in Health Care Settings," *Medical Clinics of North America* 106, no. 1 (2022): 201–217, https://linkinghub .elsevier.com/retrieve/pii/S002571252100122X.

17. "Just Say No," History.com, last updated August 21, 2018, https://www .history.com/topics/1980s/just-say-no.

18. NIH, "Harm Reduction to Lessen HIV Risks," last updated February 9, 2016, https://www.niaid.nih.gov/diseases-conditions/harm -reduction.

19. Nakagawa F et al., "Projected Life Expectancy of People with HIV According to Timing of Diagnosis," *AIDS* 26, no. 3 (2012): 335–343.

20. NIH, "HIV Undetectable=Untransmittable (U=U), or Treatment as Prevention," May 21, 2019; https://www.niaid.nih.gov/diseases -conditions/treatment-prevention.

21. Gandhi M, "The Most Important Thing Rich Countries Can Do to Help India Fight COVID-19," *Time,* May 4, 2021, https://time.com/6046096 /india-COVID-19-vaccine-patents/.

22. Chalfant M, "Biden Unveils Updated Strategy to End HIV Epidemic by 2030," *The Hill,* December 1, 2021, https://thehill.com/homenews /administration/583721-biden-unveils-updated-strategy-to-end-hiv -epidemic-by-2030/; World Health Organization, "WHO Flags Key Challenges to Global HIV Response at International AIDS Conference," July 14, 2016, https://www.who.int/news/item/14-07-2016-who-flags -key-challenges-to-global-hiv-response-at-international-aids-conference; UNAIDS, "Full Report—In Danger: UNAIDS Global AIDS Update," July 2022, https://www.unaids.org/en/resources/documents/2022 /in-danger-global-aids-update.

23. UNAIDS, "Full Report—In Danger."

24. NIH, "NIH Launches Clinical Trial of Three mRNA HIV Vaccines," March 14, 2022, https://www.nih.gov/news-events/news-releases/nih -launches-clinical-trial-three-mrna-hiv-vaccines.

25. Daignault M, Gandhi M, "The Case for Cautious COVID Optimism This Winter," *Time,* December 13, 2022, https://time.com/6240524 /covid-19-optimism-this-winter/.

26. Kofman A, Kantor R, Adashi EY, "Potential COVID-19 Endgame Scenarios: Eradication, Elimination, Cohabitation, or Conflagration?," *Journal of the American Medical Association* 326, no. 4 (2021): 303–304, https://jamanetwork.com/journals/jama/fullarticle/2781945.

27. CDC, "The Principles of Disease Elimination and Eradication," *Morbidity and Mortality Weekly Report Supplements* 48, no. SU01 (1999), https://www.cdc.gov/mmwr/preview/mmwrhtml/su48a7.htm.

28. Strassburg MA, "The Global Eradication of Smallpox," *American Journal of Infection Control* 10, no. 2 (1982): 53–59, https://linkinghub.elsevier.com/retrieve/pii/0196655382900037.

29. Griffin DE, "Measles Vaccine," *Viral Immunology* 31, no. 2 (2018): 86–95; Zucker JR et al., "Consequences of Undervaccination—Measles Outbreak, New York City, 2018–2019," *New England Journal of Medicine* 382, no. 11 (2020): 1009–1017; Marima T, Nolen S, "More Than 700 Children Have Died in a Measles Outbreak in Zimbabwe," *New York Times,* September 24, 2022, https://www.nytimes.com/2022/09/24/health/measles-outbreak-zimbabwe.html.

30. Koser T, Ruiz Aravena M, "Virulence Evolution and SARS-CoV-2/1918 H1N1 Influenza," Disease Ecology Lab, Department of Microbiology and Immunology, Montana State University, May 12, 2020, https://www.montana.edu/diseaseecologylab/COVID19blog/posts/19979/virulence-evolution-and-sars-coV-2-1918-h1n1-influenza.

31. Pickering B, "Highly Divergent White-Tailed Deer SARS-CoV-2 with Potential Deer-to-Human Transmission," *bioRxiv,* February 2022, 481551; Crist C, "COVID-19 Found in 29 Types of Animals, Scientists Say," WebMD, March 7, 2022, https://www.webmd.com/lung/news/20220307/COVID-found-in-29-types-of-animals.

32. Spinelli MA et al., "Importance of Non-Pharmaceutical Interventions in Lowering the Viral Inoculum to Reduce Susceptibility to Infection by SARS-CoV-2 and Potentially Disease Severity," *Lancet Infectious Diseases* 21, no. 9 (2021): e296–e301, https://www.thelancet.com/journals/laninf/article/PIIS1473-3099(20)30982-8/fulltext.

33. "WHO Director-General's Opening Remarks at the Media Briefing on COVID-19—11 March 2020," https://www.who.int/director-general/speeches/detail/who-director-general-s-opening-remarks-at-the-media-briefing-on-COVID-19---11-march-2020; FDA, "FDA Takes Key Action in Fight Against COVID-19 by Issuing Emergency Use Authorization for First COVID-19 Vaccine," December 11, 2020, https://www.fda.gov/news-events/press-announcements/fda-takes-key-action-fight-against-COVID-19-issuing-emergency-use-authorization-first-COVID-19.

34. Dworkin S, Gandhi M, Passano P, *Women's Empowerment and Global Health* (Berkeley: University of California Press, 2016), https://www

.ucpress.edu/book/9780520272880/womens-empowerment-and-global
-health; Sacerdote et al., "Why Is All COVID-19 News Bad News?";
Swami MK, Gupta T, "Psychological Impact of Fear-Based Messages
in Context of COVID 19," *International Journal of Social Psychiatry*
67, no. 8 (2021): 1081–1082, https://journals.sagepub.com/doi/full
/10.1177/0020764020980773.

35. Burbio, "Burbio's K–12 School Opening Tracker," 2022, https://about
.burbio.com/school-opening-tracker.

36. "Schools Should Be the Last to Close and the First to Reopen," UNICEF,
October 31, 2020, https://www.unicef.org/northmacedonia/press
-releases/schools-should-be-last-close-and-first-reopen.

37. CDC, "National Pandemic Influenza Plans," 2017, https://www.cdc
.gov/flu/pandemic-resources/planning-preparedness/national-strategy
-planning.html.

38. HHS, "U.S. Surgeon General Issues Advisory on Youth Mental Health
Crisis Further Exposed by COVID-19 Pandemic," December 7, 2021,
https://www.hhs.gov/about/news/2021/12/07/us-surgeon-general-issues
-advisory-on-youth-mental-health-crisis-further-exposed-by-COVID-19
-pandemic.html.

39. Mineo L, "Remote Learning Likely Widened Racial, Economic
Achievement Gap," *Harvard Gazette,* May 2022, https://news.harvard
.edu/gazette/story/2022/05/remote-learning-likely-widened-racial
-economic-achievement-gap/; Goldhaber D, Kane TJ, McEachin A,
Morton E, Patterson T, Staiger DO, "The Consequences of Remote
and Hybrid Instruction During the Pandemic," Working Paper No.
267-0522, National Center for the Analysis of Longitudinal Data in
Education Research, May 2022, https://caldercenter.org/publications
/consequences-remote-and-hybrid-instruction-during-pandemic.

40. George DS, "American Students' Test Scores Plunge to Levels Unseen for
Decades," *Washington Post,* September 1, 2022, https://www.washington
post.com/education/2022/09/01/student-test-scores-plunged-pandemic/.

41. AP News, "Reading and Mathematics Scores Decline During COVID-19
Pandemic," NPR, September 1, 2022, https://www.npr.org/2022/09/01
/1120510251/reading-math-test-scores-pandemic.

42. Engel FD, et al., "Impact of the COVID-19 Pandemic on the Experiences
of Hospitalized Patients: A Scoping Review," *Journal of Patient Safety*
(November 28, 2022), https://journals.lww.com/journalpatientsafety
/Fulltext/9900/Impact_of_the_COVID_19_Pandemic_on_the
_Experiences.79.aspx; Colombini S, "New Laws Let Visitors See Loved
Ones in Health Care Facilities, Even in an Outbreak," NPR, April 3,

2022, https://www.npr.org/sections/health-shots/2022/04/03/1086
216581/visiting-patients-during-COVID.

43. Swami and Gupta, "Psychological Impact of Fear-Based Messages in
Context of COVID 19."

44. Commonwealth Fund, "2022 Scorecard on State Health System
Performance: How Did States Do During the COVID-19 Pandemic?,"
June 2022, https://www.commonwealthfund.org/publications
/scorecard/2022/jun/2022-scorecard-state-health-system-performance.

45. Pulerwitz J, "How Stigma Subverts Public Health," *Nature,* November
19, 2019, https://www.nature.com/articles/d41586-019-03531-2.

46. Gandhi M, "Monkeypox and COVID: Public Health Has to Increase
Trust," *Medscape,* June 28, 2022, https://www.medscape.com/view
article/976081.

47. Pulerwitz, "How Stigma Subverts Public Health."

48. Dworkin, Gandhi, and Passano, *Women's Empowerment and Global
Health*; Eldred SM, "It's a Bleak 'Day of the Girl' Because of the
Pandemic. But No One's Giving Up Hope," NPR, October 11, 2022,
https://www.npr.org/sections/goatsandsoda/2022/10/11/1127313745
/its-a-bleak-day-of-the-girl-because-of-the-pandemic-but-no-ones-giving
-up-hope.

49. Burbio, "Burbio's K–12 School Opening Tracker."

50. California Department of Education, "Student Enrollment Reports,"
April 2022, http://www.cde.ca.gov/nr/ne/yr22/yr22rel20.asp;
Fensterwald J, Peele T, "State Delays Public Release of English, Math and
Science Test Score Results to Later This Year," EdSource, September 22,
2022, http://edsource.org/?page_id=678462; "Oregon Ranks No. 5 for
Pandemic Reading Loss, No. 8 for Math, Researchers Say," Oregon Live,
October 2022, https://www.oregonlive.com/education/2022/10/oregon
-ranks-no-5-for-pandemic-reading-loss-no-8-for-math-researchers-say
.html.

51. Broadbent A et al., "Lockdown Is Not Egalitarian: The Costs Fall on the
Global Poor," *Lancet* 396, no. 10243 (2020): 21–22, https://www.the
lancet.com/journals/lancet/article/PIIS0140-6736(20)31422-7/fulltext.

52. Robert Wood Johnson Foundation and the Harvard T.H. Chan School
of Public Health, "The Public's Perspective on the United States Public
Health System," May 13, 2021, https://cdn1.sph.harvard.edu/wp-content
/uploads/sites/94/2021/05/RWJF-Harvard-Report_FINAL-051321
.pdf; NBC News Survey, "Hart Research Associates/Public Opinion
Strategies," January 2022, https://s3.documentcloud.org/documents
/21184709/220027-nbc-news-january-poll.pdf; Gallup Poll, "Americans'

Ratings of CDC Communication Turn Negative," September 7, 2021, https://news.gallup.com/poll/354566/americans-ratings-cdc-communication-turn-negative.aspx.

53. Tram KH et al., "Deliberation, Dissent, and Distrust: Understanding Distinct Drivers of Coronavirus Disease 2019 Vaccine Hesitancy in the United States," *Clinical Infectious Diseases* 74, no. 8 (2022): 1429–1441, https://academic.oup.com/cid/article/74/8/1429/6323151; Leuchter RK et al., "Association Between COVID-19 Vaccination and Influenza Vaccination Rates," *New England Journal of Medicine* 386, no. 26 (June 2022): 2531–2532, https://www.nejm.org/doi/10.1056/NEJMc2204560; Gandhi M, "Polio Making a Comeback in the US Owing to Declining Vaccination Rates," *Medscape,* September 19, 2022, https://www.medscape.com/viewarticle/980857.

54. Stobbe M, "CDC Director Announces Shake-Up, Citing COVID Mistakes," Associated Press, August 17, 2022, https://apnews.com/article/COVID-science-health-public-rochelle-walensky-843cd83bf1d616846ff455f7f5f0d30d.

55. Appa A et al., "Drug Overdose Deaths Before and After Shelter-in-Place Orders During the COVID-19 Pandemic in San Francisco," *JAMA Network Open* 4, no. 5 (2021): e2110452, https://jamanetwork.com/journals/jamanetworkopen/fullarticle/2779782; American Medical Association, "Issue Brief: Nation's Drug-Related Overdose and Death Epidemic Continues to Worsen," September 7, 2022, https://www.ama-assn.org/system/files/issue-brief-increases-in-opioid-related-overdose.pdf.

56. San Francisco Department of Public Health, 2021 HIV Epidemiology Annual Report, September 2022, https://www.sfdph.org/dph/files/reports/RptsHIVAIDS/AnnualReport2021-Red.pdf.

57. Spinelli et al., "Importance of Non-Pharmaceutical Interventions in Lowering the Viral Inoculum to Reduce Susceptibility to Infection by SARS-CoV-2 and Potentially Disease Severity."

58. Gandhi M, "COVID-19 Vaccines Work Better and for Longer Than Expected Across Populations, Including Immunocompromised Individuals," *Medscape,* May 27, 2022, https://www.medscape.com/viewarticle/974363.

59. Gandhi M, "Want to Motivate Vaccinations? Message Optimism, Not Doom," Leaps, February 6, 2021, https://leaps.org/want-to-motivate-vaccinations-focus-on-the-reasons-for-optimism-not-continual-doom/.

60. Moore R et al., "Motivations to Vaccinate Among Hesitant Adopters of the COVID-19 Vaccine," *Journal of Community Health* 47, no. 2 (2022):

237–245, https://link.springer.com/article/10.1007/s10900-021-01037-5; Gandhi M, "The Science Is Clear: Masks Worked, but Vaccinated People Don't Need Them Now," *Washington Post,* May 18, 2021, https://www .washingtonpost.com/outlook/2021/05/18/vaccines-no-masks-cdc/.

61. Moore et al., "Motivations to Vaccinate Among Hesitant Adopters of the COVID-19 Vaccine"; Sargent RH et al., "Masks, Money, and Mandates: A National Survey on Efforts to Increase COVID-19 Vaccination Intentions in the United States," *PLoS ONE* 17, no. 4 (2022): e0267154, https://doi.org/10.1371/journal.pone.0267154.

62. Brown CM et al., "Outbreak of SARS-CoV-2 Infections, Including COVID-19 Vaccine Breakthrough Infections, Associated with Large Public Gatherings—Barnstable County, Massachusetts, July 2021," *Morbidity and Mortality Weekly Report* 70, no. 31 (2021): 1059–1062, https://www.cdc.gov/mmwr/volumes/70/wr/mm7031e2.htm.

63. Tufekci Z, "The CDC Needs to Stop Confusing the Public," *New York Times,* August 4, 2021, https://www.nytimes.com/2021/08/04/opinion /cdc-COVID-guidelines.html.

64. Yun I, "The Provincetown COVID Data Is Actually Good News (if You Are Vaccinated)," *Medium,* August 1, 2021, https://inguyun.medium .com/the-provincetown-outbreak-is-actually-good-news-if-you-are -vaccinated-93a1edd763b6.

65. Yun, "The Provincetown COVID Data Is Actually Good News (if You Are Vaccinated)"; Allsop J, "How Major Media Outlets Screwed Up the Vaccine 'Breakthrough' Story," *Columbia Journalism Review,* August 2, 2021, https://www.cjr.org/the_media_today/cdc_date_media_coverage _vaccination.php; Howard J, "CDC Updates Guidance, Recommends Vaccinated People Wear Masks Indoors in Certain Areas," CNN, July 27, 2021, https://www.cnn.com/2021/07/27/health/cdc-mask-guidance -vaccinated-people-bn.

66. Leonhardt D, "One in 5000: The Real Chances of a Breakthrough Infection," *New York Times,* September 7, 2021, https://www.nytimes .com/2021/09/07/briefing/risk-breakthrough-infections-delta.html.

67. Ng A, "Singapore Is Seeing Daily Record COVID Cases. Here's Why It May Not Be a Bad Thing," CNBC, September 27 2021, https://www .cnbc.com/2021/09/27/singapore-is-seeing-record-COVID-cases-that -may-not-be-a-bad-thing.html.

68. Chanjaroen C, "Singapore's COVID Reports Will Now Focus on Hospitalizations as Community Cases Hit Record Levels," *Fortune,* September 9, 2021, https://fortune.com/2021/09/09/singapore -COVID-hospitalized-cases-community-vaccine-rate/.

69. Harris JE, "COVID-19 Incidence and Hospitalization During the Delta Surge Were Inversely Related to Vaccination Coverage Among the Most Populous U.S. Counties," *Health Policy and Technology* 11, no. 2 (2022): 100583, https://www.sciencedirect.com/science/article/pii/S221188372 1001064; Jung Y, "Why San Francisco Is a COVID Hotspot for Cases, but Not Hospitalizations," *San Francisco Chronicle,* August 6, 2021, https://www.sfchronicle.com/health/article/The-vaccination-advantage -How-San-Francisco-s-16370752.php.

70. Harris, "COVID-19 Incidence and Hospitalization During the Delta Surge Were Inversely Related to Vaccination Coverage Among the Most Populous U.S. Counties."

71. Koenig D, "Delta Whiplash: How the New Surge Is Affecting Mental Health," WebMD, August 19, 2021, https://www.webmd.com/lung/news /20210819/delta-whiplash-how-new-surge-affecting-mental-health.

72. Gandhi M, "Don't Panic Over Waning Antibodies. Here's Why," Leaps, September 2, 2021, https://leaps.org/how-long-do-COVID-antibodies -last/.

73. Chappell B, "Here's Why Dr. Fauci Says the U.S. Is 'Out of the Pandemic Phase,'" NPR, April 28, 2022, https://www.npr.org/2022 /04/27/1094997608/fauci-us-pandemic-phase-COVID-19.

CHAPTER 2: COVID-19: HOW IT SPREAD, WHO IT AFFECTS MOST, AND HOW IT CAUSES DISEASE

1. Wade L, "From Black Death to Fatal Flu, Past Pandemics Show Why People on the Margins Suffer Most," *Science,* May 14, 2020; Amnesty International, "'There Is No Help for Our Community': The Impact of States' COVID-19 Responses on Groups Affected by Unjust Criminalization: Report," 2022, https://www.amnesty.org/en/documents /pol30/5477/2022/en/.

2. Shanks GD, Waller M, Briem H, Gottfredsson M, "Age-Specific Measles Mortality During the Late 19th–Early 20th Centuries," *Epidemiology and Infection* 143, no. 16 (2015): 3434–3441, https://doi.org/10.1017/s0950 268815000631.

3. Mehndiratta MM, Mehndiratta P, Pande R, "Poliomyelitis: Historical Facts, Epidemiology, and Current Challenges in Eradication," *Neurohospitalist* 4, no. 4 (2014): 223–229, https://doi.org/10.1177/1941 874414533352.

4. Htar TT, et al., "The Burden of Respiratory Syncytial Virus in Adults: A Systematic Review and Meta-Analysis," *Epidemiology & Infection* 148 (February 13, 2020), https://www.cambridge.org/core/journals /epidemiology-and-infection/article/burden-of-respiratory-syncytial -virus-in-adults-a-systematic-review-and-metaanalysis/B21A7EE945E9 0D98BC59C4BFB104E0E7; Shi T et al., "RSV Global Epidemiology Network. Global, Regional, and National Disease Burden Estimates of Acute Lower Respiratory Infections Due to Respiratory Syncytial Virus in Young Children in 2015: A Systematic Review and Modelling Study," *Lancet* 390, no. 10098 (September 2–8, 2017): 946–958, https://www .sciencedirect.com/science/article/pii/S0140673617309388.

5. Poehling KA, Edwards KM, Weinberg GA, et al., "The Underrecognized Burden of Influenza in Young Children," *New England Journal of Medicine* 355, no. 1 (2006): 31–40, doi:10.1056/NEJMoa054869; Talbot HK, "Influenza in Older Adults," *Infectious Disease Clinics of North America* 31, no. 4 (2017): 757–766, https://doi.org/10.1016/j.idc.2017 .07.005; Shanks GD, Brundage JF, "Pathogenic Responses Among Young Adults During the 1918 Influenza Pandemic," *Emerging Infectious Diseases* 18, no. 2 (2012): 201–207, https://doi.org/10.3201/eid1802.102042.

6. Mandavilli A, "Why the New Coronavirus (Mostly) Spares Children," *New York Times,* February 5, 2020, https://www.nytimes.com/2020/02 /05/health/coronavirus-children.html; WHO, "Report of the WHO-China Joint Mission on Coronavirus Disease 2019 (COVID-19)," 2020, https://www.who.int/publications/i/item/report-of-the-who-china-joint -mission-on-coronavirus-disease-2019-(COVID-19).

7. WHO, "COVID-19—China," 2020, https://www.who.int/emergencies /disease-outbreak-news/item/2020-DON229; WHO, "Novel Coronavirus (2019-Ncov) Situation Report—1," February 21, 2020, https://www.who.int/docs/default-source/coronaviruse/situation-reports /20200121-sitrep-1-2019-ncov.pdf.

8. V'kovski P, Kratzel A, Steiner S, Stalder H, Thiel V, "Coronavirus Biology and Replication: Implications for SARS-CoV-2," *Nature Reviews Microbiology* 19, no. 3 (2021): 155–170, doi:10.1038/ s41579-020-00468-6.

9. Gwaltney JM Jr, "Virology and Immunology of the Common Cold," *Rhinology* 23, no. 4 (1985): 265–271.

10. Berche P, "The Enigma of the 1889 Russian Flu Pandemic: A Coronavirus?," *La Presse Médicale* 51, no. 3 (2022): 104111, https://doi .org/10.1016/j.lpm.2022.104111.

11. Brüssow H, Brüssow L, "Clinical Evidence That the Pandemic from 1889 to 1891 Commonly Called the Russian Flu Might Have Been an Earlier Coronavirus Pandemic," *Microbial Biotechnology* 14, no. 5 (2021): 1860–1870, doi:10.1111/1751-7915.13889.

12. Gwaltney, "Virology and Immunology of the Common Cold."

13. Abou Ghayda, R, Lee, KH, Han, YJ, et al., "Global Case Fatality Rate of Coronavirus Disease 2019 by Continents and National Income: A Meta-Analysis," *Journal of Medical Virology* 94, no. 6 (2022), https://onlinelibrary.wiley.com/doi/10.1002/jmv.27610.

14. Gwaltney, "Virology and Immunology of the Common Cold"; Berche, "The Enigma of the 1889 Russian Flu Pandemic: A Coronavirus?"

15. Peiris JS, Yuen KY, Osterhaus AD, Stöhr K, "The Severe Acute Respiratory Syndrome," *New England Journal of Medicine* 349, no. 25 (2003): 2431–2441, doi:10.1056/NEJMra032498.

16. CDC, "CDC SARS Response Timeline," April 2013, https://www.cdc.gov/about/history/sars/timeline.htm.

17. Normile D, "SARS Found in Chinese Bats," *Science News,* September 12, 2005, https://www.science.org/content/article/sars-found-chinese-bats; Wang LF, Eaton BT, "Bats, Civets and the Emergence of SARS," in *Wildlife and Emerging Zoonotic Diseases: The Biology, Circumstances and Consequences of Cross-Species Transmission,* ed. Childs JE, Mackenzie JS, Richt JA, 325–344 (Berlin: Springer, 2007).

18. WHO, "MERS Situation Update," August 2022, https://www.emro.who.int/health-topics/mers-cov/mers-outbreaks.html.

19. Han HJ, Yu H, Yu XJ, "Evidence for Zoonotic Origins of Middle East Respiratory Syndrome Coronavirus," *Journal of General Virology* 97, no. 2 (2016): 274–280, doi:10.1099/jgv.0.000342.

20. Maxmen A, "Wuhan Market Was Epicentre of Pandemic's Start, Studies Suggest," *Nature,* February 27, 2022, https://www.nature.com/articles/d41586-022-00584-8; Zhou H, Ji J, Chen X, Bi Y, Li J, Wang Q, Hu T, et al., "Identification of Novel Bat Coronaviruses Sheds Light on the Evolutionary Origins of SARS-CoV-2 and Related Viruses," *Cell* 184, no. 17 (2021): 4380–4391.e14, https://doi.org/10.1016/j.cell.2021.06.008.

21. WHO, "Preliminary Report for the Scientific Advisory Group for the Origins of Novel Pathogens (SAGO)," 2022, https://www.who.int/publications/m/item/scientific-advisory-group-on-the-origins-of-novel-pathogens-report.

22. WHO, "WHO Coronavirus (COVID-19) Dashboard," accessed November 2022, https://COVID19.who.int/.

23. COVID-19 Excess Mortality Collaborators, "Estimating Excess Mortality Due to the COVID-19 Pandemic: A Systematic Analysis of COVID-19-Related Mortality, 2020–21," *Lancet* 399, no. 10334 (2022): 1513–1536, https://doi.org/10.1016/s0140-6736(21)02796-3.

24. Johns Hopkins University and Medicine, "Maps and Trends Mortality Analyses," accessed November 2022, https://coronavirus.jhu.edu/data/mortality.

25. Woolf SH, Chapman DA, Sabo RT, Zimmerman EB, "Excess Deaths from COVID-19 and Other Causes in the US, March 1, 2020, to January 2, 2021," *Journal of the American Medical Association* 325, no. 17 (2021): 1786–1789, https://doi.org/10.1001/jama.2021.5199.

26. "China Locks Down 21 Million Residents in Chengdu After COVID-19 Outbreak," *PBS NewsHour,* September 1, 2022, https://www.pbs.org/newshour/world/china-locks-down-21-million-residents-in-chengdu-to-after-COVID-19-outbreak.

27. Tan Y, "China Signals Ease in COVID Policy After Mass Protests," BBC News, December 1, 2022, https://www.bbc.com/news/world-asia-china-63805188.

28. CDC, "COVID Data Tracker," accessed 2022, https://COVID.cdc.gov/COVID-data-tracker/#vaccinations_vacc-people-onedose-pop-5yr; Harris JE, "COVID-19 Incidence and Hospitalization During the Delta Surge Were Inversely Related to Vaccination Coverage Among the Most Populous U.S. Counties," *Health Policy and Technology* 11, no. 2 (2022): 100583, doi:10.1016/j.hlpt.2021.100583; Schöley J, Aburto JM, Kashnitsky I, et al., "Life Expectancy Changes Since COVID-19," *Nature Human Behaviour,* October 17, 2022, https://doi.org/10.1038/s41562-022-01450-3; Flam F, "The Tragedy of Avoidable COVID Deaths," Bloomberg, December 3, 2022, https://www.bloomberg.com/opinion/articles/2022-12-03/low-us-COVID-vaccine-rates-led-to-high-death-rates-during-delta-omicron?srnd=premium-europe.

29. Schöley et al., "Life Expectancy Changes Since COVID-19."

30. Bilinski A, Thompson K, Emanuel E, "COVID-19 and Excess All-Cause Mortality in the US and 20 Comparison Countries, June 2021–March 2022," *Journal of the American Medical Association* (online), November 18, 2022, doi:10.1001/jama.2022.21795; Flam, "The Tragedy of Avoidable COVID Deaths."

31. Dykgraaf SH, Matenge S, Desborough J, Sturgiss E, Dut G, Roberts L, McMillan A, Kidd M, "Protecting Nursing Homes and Long-Term Care Facilities from COVID-19: A Rapid Review of International Evidence," *JAMDA: The Journal of Post-Acute and Long-Term Care Medicine* 22,

no. 10 (2021): 1969–1988, https://doi.org/10.1016/j.jamda.2021.07.027;
Preskorn SH, "The 5% of the Population at High Risk for Severe
COVID-19 Infection Is Identifiable and Needs to Be Taken into Account
When Reopening the Economy," *Journal of Psychiatric Practice* 26, no. 3
(2020): 219–227, https://doi.org/10.1097/pra.0000000000000475.

32. Tai DBG, Sia IG, Doubeni CA, Wieland ML, "Disproportionate Impact
of COVID-19 on Racial and Ethnic Minority Groups in the United
States: A 2021 Update," *Journal of Racial and Ethnic Health Disparities* 9
(2022): 2334–2339, https://doi.org/10.1007/s40615-021-01170-w;
Crist C, "COVID Death Rate for White Americans Now Exceeds
Others: Report," WebMD, June 9, 2022, https://www.webmd.com/lung
/news/20220609/COVID-death-rate-white-americans-exceeds-others
-report.

33. Price-Haywood EG, Burton J, Fort D, Seoane L, "Hospitalization and
Mortality Among Black Patients and White Patients with COVID-19,"
New England Journal of Medicine 382, no. 26 (2020): 2534–2543,
doi:10.1056/NEJMsa2011686.

34. "How the Race Gap in COVID-19 Deaths Flipped," *All Things
Considered,* NPR, October 29, 2022, https://www.npr.org/2022/10/29
/1132633496/how-the-race-gap-in-COVID-19-deaths-flipped.

35. Hamad R, Galea S, "The Role of Health Care Systems in Bolstering
the Social Safety Net to Address Health Inequities in the Wake of the
COVID-19 Pandemic," *Journal of the American Medical Association* 328,
no. 1 (2022): 17–18, doi:10.1001/jama.2022.10160; OECD, "Paid Sick
Leave to Protect Income, Health and Jobs Through the COVID-19
Crisis," 2020, https://www.oecd.org/coronavirus/policy-responses/paid
-sick-leave-to-protect-income-health-and-jobs-through-the-COVID-19
-crisis-a9e1a154/.

36. Galvani AP, Parpia AS, Pandey A, et al., "Universal Healthcare as
Pandemic Preparedness: The Lives and Costs That Could Have Been
Saved During the COVID-19 Pandemic," *Proceedings of the National
Academy of Sciences* 119, no. 25 (2022): e2200536119, doi:10.1073
/pnas.2200536119.

37. Li Y, Qian H, Hang J, Chen X, Cheng P, Ling H, Wang S, et al.,
"Probable Airborne Transmission of SARS-CoV-2 in a Poorly Ventilated
Restaurant," *Building and Environment* 196 (2021): 107788, https://doi
.org/10.1016/j.buildenv.2021.107788.

38. Meister TL, Dreismeier M, Blanco EV, Brüggemann Y, Heinen N,
Kampf G, Todt D, et al., "Low Risk of SARS-CoV-2 Transmission
by Fomites—a Clinical Observational Study in Highly Infectious

COVID-19 Patients," *Journal of Infectious Diseases* 226, no. 9 (2022): 1608–1615, https://doi.org/10.1093/infdis/jiac170.

39. Zhu Y, Oishi W, Maruo C, Saito M, Chen R, Kitajima M, Sano D, "Early Warning of COVID-19 Via Wastewater-Based Epidemiology: Potential and Bottlenecks," *Science of the Total Environment* 767 (2021): 145124, https://doi.org/10.1016/j.scitotenv.2021.145124.

40. Buitrago-Garcia D, et al., "Occurrence and Transmission Potential of Asymptomatic and Presymptomatic SARS-CoV-2 Infections: A Living Systematic Review and Meta-Analysis," *PLOS Medicine* 17, no. 9 (2020): e1003346, https://doi.org/10.1371/journal.pmed.1003346.

41. Qian H, Miao T, Liu L, Zheng X, Luo D, Li Y, "Indoor Transmission of SARS-CoV-2," *Indoor Air* 31, no. 3 (2021): 639–645, https://doi.org/10.1111/ina.12766.

42. White House, "Biden Administration Launches Effort to Improve Ventilation and Reduce the Spread of COVID-19 in Buildings," March 17, 2022, https://www.whitehouse.gov/briefing-room/statements-releases/2022/03/17/fact-sheet-biden-administration-launches-effort-to-improve-ventilation-and-reduce-the-spread-of-COVID-19-in-buildings/.

43. Carleton T, Cornetet J, Huybers P, Meng KC, Proctor J, "Global Evidence for Ultraviolet Radiation Decreasing COVID-19 Growth Rates," *Proceedings of the National Academy of Sciences* 118, no. 1 (2021): e2012370118, https://doi.org/10.1073/pnas.2012370118.

44. Jones TC, Biele G, Mühlemann B, et al., "Estimating Infectiousness Throughout SARS-CoV-2 Infection Course," *Science* 373, no. 6551 (2021): eabi5273, doi:10.1126/science.abi5273.

45. Cevik M, Tate M, Lloyd O, Maraolo AE, Schafers J, Ho A, "SARS-CoV-2, SARS-CoV, and MERS-CoV Viral Load Dynamics, Duration of Viral Shedding, and Infectiousness: A Systematic Review and Meta-Analysis," *Lancet Microbe* 2, no. 1 (2021): e13–e22, https://doi.org/10.1016/s2666-5247(20)30172-5.

46. Jung J, Kim JY, Park H, et al., "Transmission and Infectious SARS-CoV-2 Shedding Kinetics in Vaccinated and Unvaccinated Individuals," *JAMA Network Open* 5, no. 5 (2022): e2213606, doi:10.1001/jamanetworkopen.2022.13606.

47. Cheng HY, Jian SW, Liu DP, Ng TC, Huang WT, Lin HH, and the Taiwan COVID-19 Outbreak Investigation Team, "Contact Tracing Assessment of COVID-19 Transmission Dynamics in Taiwan and Risk at Different Exposure Periods Before and After Symptom Onset," *JAMA Internal Medicine* 180, no. 9 (2020): 1156–1163, https://doi.org/10.1001/jamainternmed.2020.2020; CDC, "CDC Updates and Shortens

Recommended Isolation and Quarantine Period for General Population," December 27, 2021, https://www.cdc.gov/media/releases/2021/s1227 -isolation-quarantine-guidance.html.

48. Faulkner D, "COVID: End of Legal Need to Self-Isolate in England," BBC News, February 24, 2022, https://www.bbc.com/news/uk-605 00287.

49. Taylor CA, Patel K, Pham H, Whitaker M, Anglin O, Kambhampati AK, Milucky J, et al., "Severity of Disease Among Adults Hospitalized with Laboratory-Confirmed COVID-19 Before and During the Period of SARS-CoV-2 B.1.617.2 (Delta) Predominance—COVID-Net, 14 States, January–August 2021," *Morbidity and Mortality Weekly Report* 70, no. 43 (2021): 1513–1519, https://doi.org/10.15585/mmwr.mm70 43e1.

50. Lewnard JA, Hong VX, Patel MM, Kahn R, Lipsitch M, Tartof SY, "Clinical Outcomes Associated with SARS-CoV-2 Omicron (B.1.1.529) Variant and Ba.1/Ba.1.1 or Ba.2 Subvariant Infection in Southern California," *Nature Medicine* 28, no. 9 (2022): 1933–1943, https:// doi.org/10.1038/s41591-022-01887-z; Nyberg T, et al., "Comparative Analysis of the Risks of Hospitalisation and Death Associated with SARS-CoV-2 Omicron (B.1.1.529) and Delta (B.1.617.2) Variants in England: A Cohort Study," *Lancet* 399, no. 10332 (April 2022): 1303– 1312, https://www.sciencedirect.com/science/article/pii/S014067362 2004627.

51. Tarke A, Coelho CH, Zhang Z, Dan JM, Yu ED, Methot N, Bloom NI, et al., "SARS-CoV-2 Vaccination Induces Immunological T Cell Memory Able to Cross-Recognize Variants from Alpha to Omicron," *Cell* 185, no. 5 (2022): 847–859.e11, https://doi.org/10.1016/j.cell.2022.01.015.

52. Murray C, "COVID-19 Will Continue but the End of the Pandemic Is Near," *Lancet* 399, no. 10323 (2022): P417–419, https://www .thelancet.com/journals/lancet/article/PIIS0140-6736(22)00100-3 /fulltext.

53. Oran DP, Topol EJ, "The Proportion of SARS-CoV-2 Infections That Are Asymptomatic: A Systematic Review," *Annals of Internal Medicine* 174, no. 5 (2021): 655–662, https://doi.org/10.7326/m20-6976; Joung SY, et al., "Awareness of SARS-CoV-2 Omicron Variant Infection Among Adults with Recent COVID-19 Seropositivity," *JAMA Network Open* 5, no. 8 (August 2022): e2227241, https://jamanetwork.com/journals /jamanetworkopen/fullarticle/2795246.

54. Johansson M, Quandelacy TM, Kada S, Prasad PV, Steele M, Brooks JT, Slayton RB, Biggerstaff M, Butler JC, "SARS-CoV-2 Transmission from

People Without COVID-19 Symptoms," *JAMA Network Open* 4, no. 1 (2021): e2035057-e57, https://doi.org/10.1001/jamanetworkopen.2020 .35057.

55. Buitrago-Garcia et al., "Occurrence and Transmission Potential."

56. Cohen C, Kleynhans J, Moyes J, McMorrow ML, Treurnicht FK, Hellferscee O, Mathunjwa A, et al., "Asymptomatic Transmission and High Community Burden of Seasonal Influenza in an Urban and a Rural Community in South Africa, 2017–18 (Phirst): A Population Cohort Study," *Lancet Global Health* 9, no. 6 (2021): e863–e874, https://doi .org/10.1016/s2214-109x(21)00141-8.

57. Department of Health and Social Care, UK, "Regular Asymptomatic Testing Paused in Additional Settings," news release, 2022, https://www .gov.uk/government/news/regular-asymptomatic-testing-paused-in -additional-settings.

58. CDC, "Interim Infection Prevention and Control Recommendations for Healthcare Personnel During the Coronavirus Disease 2019 (COVID-19) Pandemic," last updated September 23, 2022, https://www.cdc.gov /coronavirus/2019-ncov/hcp/infection-control-recommendations.html.

59. Binnicker MJ, "Can Testing Predict SARS-CoV-2 Infectivity? The Potential for Certain Methods to Be Surrogates for Replication-Competent Virus," *Journal of Clinical Microbiology* 59, no. 11 (2021): e0046921, doi:10.1128/JCM.00469-21.

60. Connor BA, Rogova M, Garcia J, et al., "Comparative Effectiveness of Single vs Repeated Rapid SARS-CoV-2 Antigen Testing Among Asymptomatic Individuals in a Workplace Setting," *JAMA Network Open* 5, no. 3 (2022): e223073, doi:10.1001/jamanetworkopen.2022.3073.

61. Wu Z, McGoogan JM, "Characteristics of and Important Lessons from the Coronavirus Disease 2019 (COVID-19) Outbreak in China: Summary of a Report of 72,314 Cases from the Chinese Center for Disease Control and Prevention," *Journal of the American Medical Association* 323, no. 13 (2020): 1239–1242, doi:10.1001/jama.2020.2648.

62. Menni C, Valdes AM, Polidori L, et al., "Symptom Prevalence, Duration, and Risk of Hospital Admission in Individuals Infected with SARS-CoV-2 During Periods of Omicron and Delta Variant Dominance: A Prospective Observational Study from the ZOE COVID Study," *Lancet* 399, no. 10335 (2022): 1618–1624, doi:10.1016/S0140-6736(22)0 0327-0.

63. Mallapaty S, "Kids and COVID: Why Young Immune Systems Are Still on Top," *Nature,* September 7, 2021, https://www.nature.com/articles /d41586-021-02423-8.

64. Mueller B, "Despite Another COVID Surge, Deaths Stay Near Lows," *New York Times,* June 20, 2022, https://www.nytimes.com/2022/06/20 /health/COVID-deaths-plateau.html.

65. Jassat W, et al., "Trends in Cases, Hospitalization and Mortality Related to the Omicron BA.4/BA.5 Sub-Variants in South Africa," *Clinical Infectious Diseases* (December 2022), https://academic.oup.com/cid /advance-article/doi/10.1093/cid/ciac921/6855554.

66. COVID-19 Forecasting Team, "Variation in the COVID-19 Infection-Fatality Ratio by Age, Time, and Geography During the Pre-Vaccine Era: A Systematic Analysis," *Lancet* 399, no. 10334 (2022): 1469–1488, doi:10.1016/S0140-6736(21)02867-1 (published correction appears in *Lancet* 399, no. 10334 (2022): 1468).

67. Lewnard et al., "Clinical Outcomes Associated with SARS-CoV-2 Omicron (B.1.1.529) Variant and Ba.1/Ba.1.1 or Ba.2 Subvariant Infection in Southern California."

68. Yek C, Warner S, Wiltz JL, et al., "Risk Factors for Severe COVID-19 Outcomes Among Persons Aged ≥18 Years Who Completed a Primary COVID-19 Vaccination Series—465 Health Care Facilities, United States, December 2020–October 2021," *Morbidity and Mortality Weekly Report* 71, no. 1 (January 7, 2022): 19–25, http://dx.doi.org/10.15585 /mmwr.mm7101a4.

69. Arbel R, Wolff Sagy Y, Hoshen M, et al., "Nirmatrelvir Use and Severe COVID-19 Outcomes During the Omicron Surge," *New England Journal of Medicine* 387, no. 9 (2022):790–798, doi:10.1056/NEJMoa2204919.

70. Agrawal U, Bedston S, McCowan C, et al., "Severe COVID-19 Outcomes After Full Vaccination of Primary Schedule and Initial Boosters: Pooled Analysis of National Prospective Cohort Studies of 30 Million Individuals in England, Northern Ireland, Scotland, and Wales," *Lancet* 400, no. 10360 (2022): 1305–1320, doi: 10.1016/S0140-6736 (22)01656-7.

71. Doron S, Gandhi M, "New Boosters Are Here! Who Should Receive Them and When?," *Lancet Infectious Diseases* (online), October 27, 2022, https://doi.org/10.1016/S1473-3099(22)00688-0; Arbel et al., "Nirmatrelvir Use and Severe COVID-19 Outcomes During the Omicron Surge."

72. Huang L, Yao Q, Gu X, et al., "1-Year Outcomes in Hospital Survivors with COVID-19: A Longitudinal Cohort Study," *Lancet* 398, no. 10302 (2021): 747–758, doi:10.1016/S0140-6736(21)01755-4.

73. Radtke T, Ulyte A, Puhan MA, Kriemler S, "Long-Term Symptoms After SARS-CoV-2 Infection in Children and Adolescents," *Journal of the*

American Medical Association 326, no. 9 (2021): 869–871, doi:10.1001
/jama.2021.11880; Nalbandian A, Sehgal K, Gupta A, et al., "Post-Acute
COVID-19 Syndrome," *Nature Medicine* 27, no. 4 (2021): 601–615,
doi:10.1038/s41591-021-01283-z.

74. Sneller MC, Liang CJ, Marques AR, et al., "A Longitudinal Study of
COVID-19 Sequelae and Immunity: Baseline Findings," *Annals of
Internal Medicine* 175, no. 7 (2022): 969–979, doi:10.7326/M21-4905.

75. Wessely S et al., "Postinfectious Fatigue: Prospective Cohort Study in
Primary Care," *Lancet* 345, no. 8961 (May 27, 1995): 1333–1338, https://
linkinghub.elsevier.com/retrieve/pii/S0140673695925376; Wisk LE et al.,
"Association of Initial SARS-CoV-2 Test Positivity with Patient-Reported
Well-Being 3 Months After a Symptomatic Illness," *JAMA Network Open*
5, no. 12 (December 1, 2022): e2244486, https://jamanetwork.com/
journals/jamanetworkopen/fullarticle/2799116.

76. Kuodi P, Gorelik Y, Zayyad H, et al., "Association Between BNT162b2
Vaccination and Reported Incidence of Post-COVID-19 Symptoms:
Cross-Sectional Study 2020–21, Israel," *NPJ Vaccines* 7, no. 1 (2022):
101, doi:10.1038/s41541-022-00526-5; Kreier F, "Long-COVID
Symptoms Less Likely in Vaccinated People, Israeli Data Say," *Nature
News,* January 25, 2022, https://www.nature.com/articles/d41586-022
-00177-5.

77. Nalbandian et al., "Post-Acute COVID-19 Syndrome"; Global Burden of
Disease Long COVID Collaborators, "Estimated Global Proportions of
Individuals with Persistent Fatigue, Cognitive, and Respiratory Symptom
Clusters Following Symptomatic COVID-19 in 2020 and 2021," *Journal
of the American Medical Association* 328, no. 16 (2022): 1604–1615,
doi:10.1001/jama.2022.18931.

78. Block J, "COVID-19: US Tracker Overestimated Deaths Among
Children," *BMJ* 376 (2022): o831, doi:10.1136/bmj.o831; Mandavilli
A, "The C.D.C. Isn't Publishing Large Portions of the COVID Data It
Collects," *New York Times,* February 20, 2022, https://www.nytimes
.com/2022/02/20/health/COVID-cdc-data.html; Kelley, "What's
Wrong with CDC Data on Pediatric Mortality?," COVID-19 in Georgia,
accessed 2021, https://www.COVID-georgia.com/pediatric-news
/whats-wrong-with-cdc-data-on-pediatric-mortality/.

79. Bertran M, Amin-Chowdhury Z, Davies H, et al., "COVID-19 Deaths
in Children and Young People: Active Prospective National Surveillance,
March 2020 to December 2021, England," *PLOS Medicine* 19, no. 11
(November 8, 2022): e1004118, https://journals.plos.org/plosmedicine
/article?id=10.1371/journal.pmed.1004118.

80. Office of National Statistics (UK), "Coronavirus (COVID-19) Latest Insights: Deaths," October 2022, https://www.ons.gov.uk /peoplepopulationandcommunity/healthandsocialcare/conditions anddiseases/articles/coronavirusCOVID19latestinsights/deaths.

81. Haigh KZ, Gandhi M, "COVID-19 Mitigation with Appropriate Safety Measures in an Essential Workplace: Lessons for Opening Work Settings in the United States During COVID-19," *Open Forum Infectious Diseases* 8, no. 4 (2021): ofab086, doi:10.1093/ofid/ofab086.

82. White House, "Biden Administration Launches Effort to Improve Ventilation and Reduce the Spread of COVID-19 in Buildings."

83. Simon J, Helter TM, White RG, van der Boor C, Łaszewska A, "Impacts of the COVID-19 Lockdown and Relevant Vulnerabilities on Capability Well-Being, Mental Health and Social Support: An Austrian Survey Study," *BMC Public Health* 21, no. 1 (2021): 314, doi:10.1186 /s12889-021-10351-5; Mahler D, Yonzan N, Lakner C, et al., "Updated Estimates of the Impact of COVID-19 on Global Poverty: Turning the Corner on the Pandemic in 2021?," World Bank *Data Blog,* June 24, 2021, https://blogs.worldbank.org/opendata/updated -estimates-impact-COVID-19-global-poverty-turning-corner-pandemic -2021; UNICEF, "UNICEF: An Additional 6.7 Million Children Under 5 Could Suffer from Wasting This Year Due to COVID-19," press release, July 27, 2020, https://www.unicef.org/press-releases/unicef -additional-67-million-children-under-5-could-suffer-wasting-year -due-COVID-19; Lipman M, McQuaid CF, Abubakar I, Khan M, Kranzer K, McHugh TD, Padmapriyadarsini C, Rangaka MX, Stoker N, "The Impact of COVID-19 on Global Tuberculosis Control," *Indian Journal of Medical Research* 153, no. 4 (2021): 404–408, https://doi.org/10.4103/ijmr.IJMR_326_21; Zawawi A, Alghanmi M, Alsaady I, Gattan H, Zakai H, Couper K, "The Impact of COVID-19 Pandemic on Malaria Elimination," *Parasite Epidemiology and Control* 11 (2020): e00187, doi:10.1016/j.parepi.2020 .e00187; Dorward J, Khubone T, Gate K, et al., "The Impact of the COVID-19 Lockdown on HIV Care in 65 South African Primary Care Clinics: An Interrupted Time Series Analysis," *Lancet HIV* 8, no. 3 (2021): e158–e165, doi:10.1016/S2352-3018(20)30359-3; Gandhi M, "Global HIV Goals Suffer Major Setbacks During COVID-19, According to UNAIDS Report for 2022," *Medscape,* August 22, 2022, https://www.medscape.com/viewarticle/979292; Patt D, "Impact of COVID-19 on Cancer Care: How the Pandemic Is Delaying

Cancer Diagnosis and Treatment for American Seniors," *JCO Clinical Care Informatics* 4 (November 30, 2020), https://ascopubs.org/doi/full/10.1200/CCI.20.00134; "COVID-19 Pandemic Indirectly Disrupted Heart Disease Care," American College of Cardiology, January 11, 2021, https://www.acc.org/about-acc/press-releases/2021/01/11/16/40/COVID19-pandemic-indirectly-disrupted-heart-disease-care; Kuehn B, "CDC Report: Urgent Need to Address Teens' Adverse Experiences During Pandemic," *JAMA* 328, no. 20 (November 22/29, 2022): 2005, https://jamanetwork.com/journals/jama/fullarticle/2798730.

84. "10 Killed in Apartment Fire in China's Xinjiang," CBS News, November 25, 2022, https://www.cbsnews.com/news/10-killed-in-apartment-fire-in-chinas-xinjiang/; Yeung J, et al., "How a Deadly Fire Ignited Dissent over China's Zero-COVID Policy," CNN, December 3, 2022, https://www.cnn.com/2022/12/02/china/china-COVID-lockdown-protests-2022-intl-hnk-dst/index.html; Tan, "China Signals Ease in COVID Policy After Mass Protests."

85. Diamond D, "Mask Mandates Make a Return—Along with Controversy," *Washington Post,* July 19, 2021, https://www.washingtonpost.com/health/2021/07/19/mask-mandates-returning/.

86. Gandhi M, Havlir D, "The Time for Universal Masking of the Public for Coronavirus Disease 2019 Is Now," *Open Forum Infectious Diseases* 7, no. 4 (2020): ofaa131, doi:10.1093/ofid/ofaa131.

87. Gandhi M, Rutherford GW, "Facial Masking for COVID-19—Potential for 'Variolation' as We Await a Vaccine," *New England Journal of Medicine* 383, no. 18 (2020): e101, doi:10.1056/NEJMp2026913.

88. Martín-Sánchez M, Lim WW, Yeung A, et al., "COVID-19 Transmission in Hong Kong Despite Universal Masking," *Journal of Infection* 83, no. 1 (2021): 92–95, doi:10.1016/j.jinf.2021.04.019.

89. Hofer U, "Dose-Dependent COVID-19 Symptoms," *Nature Reviews Microbiology* 19, no. 11 (2021): 682, doi:10.1038/s41579-021-00634-4.

90. NIH, "Researchers Propose That Humidity from Masks May Lessen Severity of COVID-19," press release, February 12, 2021, https://www.nih.gov/news-events/news-releases/researchers-propose-humidity-masks-may-lessen-severity-COVID-19.

91. Abaluck J, Kwong LH, Styczynski A, et al., "Impact of Community Masking on COVID-19: A Cluster-Randomized Trial in Bangladesh," *Science* 375, no. 6577 (2022): eabi9069, doi:10.1126/science.abi9069.

92. Chikina M, Pegden W, Recht B, "Re-Analysis on the Statistical Sampling Biases of a Mask Promotion Trial in Bangladesh: A Statistical Replication," *Trials* 23, no. 1 (2022): 786, doi:10.1186/s13063-022 -06704-z.

93. Anderson J, "Do Masks Work? A Review of the Evidence," *City Journal*, August 11, 2021, https://www.city-journal.org/do-masks-work-a-review -of-the-evidence; Bundgaard H, et al., "Effectiveness of Adding a Mask Recommendation to Other Public Health Measures to Prevent SARS-CoV-2 Infection in Danish Mask Wearers: A Randomized Controlled Trial," *Annals of Internal Medicine* 174, no. 3 (March 2021): 335–343, https://www.acpjournals.org/doi/10.7326/M20-6817.

94. Flam F, "Mask Mandates Didn't Make Much of a Difference Anyway," Bloomberg, February 11, 2022, https://www.bloomberg.com/opinion /articles/2022-02-11/did-mask-mandates-work-the-data-is-in-and-the -answer-is-no; Leonhardt D, "Why Masks Work, but Mandates Haven't," *New York Times*, May 31, 2022, https://www.nytimes.com/2022/05/31 /briefing/masks-mandates-us-COVID.html; Guerra D, Guerra DJ, "Mask Mandate and Use Efficacy for COVID-19 Containment in US States," *medRxiv*, August 7, 2021, https://doi.org/10.1101/2021.05 .18.21257385; Schauer SG, Naylor JF, April MD, Carius BM, Hudson IL, "Analysis of the Effects of COVID-19 Mask Mandates on Hospital Resource Consumption and Mortality at the County Level," *Southern Medical Journal* 114, no. 9 (2021): 597–602, https://doi.org/10.14423 /SMJ.0000000000001294.

95. Ting E, "California Mask Mandates Are Back amid Omicron's Rise. Here's How Well They Fared vs. Delta," SFGate, December 15, 2021, https://www.sfgate.com/california-politics/article/California-mask -mandate-omicron-16701224.php.

96. Tan ST, et al., "Infectiousness of SARS-CoV-2 Breakthrough Infections and Reinfections During the Omicron Wave," *medRxiv*, November 21, 2022, https://doi.org/10.1101/2022.08.08.22278547.

97. CDC, "Prioritizing Case Investigation and Contact Tracing for COVID-19," February 28, 2022, https://www.cdc.gov/coronavirus/2019 -ncov/php/contact-tracing/contact-tracing-plan/prioritization.html.

98. Meredith GR, Diel DG, Frazier PI, et al., "Routine Surveillance and Vaccination on a University Campus During the Spread of the SARS-CoV-2 Omicron Variant," *JAMA Network Open* 5, no. 5 (2022): e2212906, doi:10.1001/jamanetworkopen.2022.12906.

99. Leonhardt, "Why Masks Work, but Mandates Haven't."

100. Khazan O, "One-Way Masking Works," *The Atlantic,* January 10, 2022, https://www.theatlantic.com/politics/archive/2022/01/does-it-help-wear-mask-if-no-one-else/621177/.

101. Behsudi A, "Denmark's Social Trust in Action," International Monetary Fund, February 2, 2022, https://www.imf.org/en/News/Articles/2022/02/01/cf-denmark-social-trust-in-action.

102. Smelkinson M, Bienen L, Noble J, "The Case Against Masks at School," *The Atlantic,* January 26, 2022, https://www.theatlantic.com/ideas/archive/2022/01/kids-masks-schools-weak-science/621133/.

103. Coma E, Català M, Méndez-Boo L, et al., "Unravelling the Role of the Mandatory Use of Face Covering Masks for the Control of SARS-CoV-2 in Schools: A Quasi-Experimental Study Nested in a Population-Based Cohort in Catalonia (Spain)," *Archives of Disease in Childhood* (online), August 23, 2022, doi:10.1136/archdischild-2022-324172.

104. WHO, "Coronavirus Disease (COVID-19): Children and Masks," March 7, 2022, https://www.who.int/news-room/questions-and-answers/item/q-a-children-and-masks-related-to-COVID-19; Ludvigsson JF, Engerström L, Nordenhäll C, Larsson E, "Open Schools, COVID-19, and Child and Teacher Morbidity in Sweden," *New England Journal of Medicine* 384, no. 7 (2021): 669–671, doi:10.1056/NEJMc2026670.

105. Charney SA, Camarata SM, Chern A, "Potential Impact of the COVID-19 Pandemic on Communication and Language Skills in Children," *Otolaryngology—Head and Neck Surgery* 165, no. 1 (2021): 1–2, doi:10.1177/0194599820978247.

106. Hughes RC, Bhopal SS, Tomlinson M, "Making Pre-School Children Wear Masks Is Bad Public Health," *Public Health in Practice* 2 (2021): 100197, doi:10.1016/j.puhip.2021.100197; Charney et al., "Potential Impact of the COVID-19 Pandemic on Communication and Language Skills in Children."

107. Gunaratne L, "Visual Impairment: Its Effect on Cognitive Development and Behaviour," University of Hertfordshire, 2002, http://www.intellectualdisability.info/physical-health/articles/visual-impairment-its-effect-on-cognitive-development-and-behaviour.

108. Frota S, Pejovic J, Cruz M, Severino C, Vigário M, "Early Word Segmentation Behind the Mask," *Frontiers in Psychology* 13 (2022): 879123, doi:10.3389/fpsyg.2022.879123.

109. Chester M, Plate RC, et al., "The COVID-19 Pandemic, Mask-Wearing, and Emotion Recognition During Late-Childhood," *Social Development,*

August 25, 2022, https://onlinelibrary.wiley.com/doi/10.1111/sode
.12631.

110. Office for Standards in Education, Children's Services and Skills (UK),
"Strong Signs of Recovery Across Education, but Challenges Remain,"
press release, April 4, 2022, https://www.gov.uk/government/news
/strong-signs-of-recovery-across-education-but-challenges-remain.

111. Byrne S, Sledge H, Franklin R, et al., "Social Communication Skill
Attainment in Babies Born During the COVID-19 Pandemic: A Birth
Cohort Study," *Archives of Disease in Childhood* (online), October 11,
2022, doi:10.1136/archdischild-2021-323441.

112. Steenhuysen J, Roy M, "WHO Lays Out Plan to Emerge from
Emergency Phase of Pandemic," Reuters, March 30, 2022, https://www
.reuters.com/business/healthcare-pharmaceuticals/who-lays-out-plan
-emerge-emergency-phase-pandemic-2022-03-30/; Pronczuk M, "The
European Union Says the Emergency Phase of the Pandemic Is Over,"
New York Times, April 27, 2022, https://www.nytimes.com/2022/04/27
/world/european-union-COVID.html; Achenbach J, Pietsch B, "U.S. No
Longer in 'Full-Blown' Pandemic Phase, Fauci Says," *Washington Post,*
April 27, 2022, https://www.washingtonpost.com/health/2022/04/27
/pandemic-phase-over-fauci-COVID/.

113. Massetti GM, Jackson BR, Brooks JT, et al., "Summary of Guidance
for Minimizing the Impact of COVID-19 on Individual Persons,
Communities, and Health Care Systems—United States," *Morbidity and
Mortality Weekly Report* 71, no. 33 (2022): 1057–1064, http://dx.doi
.org/10.15585/mmwr.mm7133e1.

114. Chandra A, Høeg TB, "Lack of Correlation Between School Mask
Mandates and Paediatric COVID-19 Cases in a Large Cohort," *Journal of
Infection* (online), September 29, 2022, https://doi.org/10.1016/j.jinf
.2022.09.019; Ladhani SN, "Face Masking for Children—Time
to Reconsider," *Journal of Infection* (online), September 25, 2022,
doi:10.1016/j.jinf.2022.09.020.

115. "Face Coverings Have Little Utility for Young School-Aged Children,"
Archives of Disease in Childhood, November 23, 2022 (epub ahead of
publication), https://adc.bmj.com/content/early/2022/11/03/archdis
child-2022-324809.

116. Steenhuysen and Roy, "WHO Lays Out Plan to Emerge from Emergency
Phase of Pandemic."

117. Pronczuk, "The European Union Says the Emergency Phase of the
Pandemic Is Over."

118. Massetti et al., "Summary of Guidance for Minimizing the Impact of COVID-19 on Individual Persons, Communities, and Health Care Systems—United States."

119. WHO, "The End of the COVID-19 Pandemic Is in Sight: WHO," September 14, 2022, https://news.un.org/en/story/2022/09/1126621.

120. Emanuel EJ, Osterholm M, Gounder CR, "A National Strategy for the 'New Normal' of Life with COVID," *Journal of the American Medical Association* 327, no. 3 (2022): 211–212, doi:10.1001/jama.2021.24282.

CHAPTER 3: HOW DO WE
MANAGE COVID-19 NOW?

1. Gandhi M, "We Won't Eradicate COVID-19. The Pandemic Will Still End," *Washington Post,* September 21, 2021, https://www.washington post.com/outlook/2021/09/21/COVID-pandemic-end/.

2. Crist C, "COVID-19 Found in 29 Types of Animals, Scientists Say," WebMD, March 7, 2022, https://www.webmd.com/lung/news/2022 0307/COVID-found-in-29-types-of-animals.

3. Kesslen B, "Here's Why Denmark Killed 17 Million Minks After More Than 200 COVID Outbreaks at Fur Farm," NBC News, December 1, 2020, https://www.nbcnews.com/news/animal-news/here-s-why -denmark-culled-17-million-minks-now-plans-n1249610; Mahtani S, Yu T, "Hong Kong Hamster Massacre: Residents Resist 'Zero COVID' City's Pet Project," *Washington Post,* January 20, 2022, https://www .washingtonpost.com/world/2022/01/20/hong-kong-hamsters-COVID/; Yeung J, "Shanghai COVID-19: Video Shows Health Worker Beating Dog to Death After Owner Tests Positive," CNN, April 8, 2022, https:// www.cnn.com/2022/04/08/china/shanghai-corgi-death-china-COVID -intl-hnk/index.html.

4. Haworth J, "8 Big Cats Confirmed Tested Positive for Coronavirus at NY Zoo," ABC News, April 23, 2020, https://abcnews.go.com/US/big -cats-test-positive-COVID-19-zookeeper-accidentally/story?id=7030 3070.

5. National Center for Biotechnology Information, "Severe Acute Respiratory Syndrome Coronavirus 2 Isolate Wuhan-Hu-1, Complete Genome," NCBI Nucleotide Database 1798172431, no. 3, March 2020, http://www.ncbi.nlm.nih.gov/nuccore/MN908947.3.

6. Korber B, Fischer WM, Gnanakaran S, et al., "Tracking Changes in SARS-CoV-2 Spike: Evidence That D614G Increases Infectivity of the COVID-19 Virus," *Cell* 182, no. 4 (2020): 812–827.e19, https://doi:10.1016/j.cell.2020.06.043.

7. Global Virus Network, "Beta (B.1.351)," February 2021, https://gvn.org/COVID-19/beta-b-1-351/; Banho CA, Sacchetto L, Campos GRF, et al., "Impact of SARS-CoV-2 Gamma Lineage Introduction and COVID-19 Vaccination on the Epidemiological Landscape of a Brazilian City," *Communications Medicine* 2, no. 1 (2022): 41, https://doi:10.1038/s43856-022-00108-5.

8. Taylor CA, Patel K, Pham H, et al., "Severity of Disease Among Adults Hospitalized with Laboratory-Confirmed COVID-19 Before and During the Period of SARS-CoV-2 B.1.617.2 (Delta) Predominance—COVID-NET, 14 States, January–August 2021," *Morbidity and Mortality Weekly Report* 70, no. 43 (2021): 1513–1519, http://doi.org/10.15585/mmwr.mm7043e1; McGregor G, Mukherji B, Mellor S, "Delta Waves in India and the U.K. Have Already Receded. Could the Same Happen in the U.S.?," *Fortune*, August 3, 2021, https://fortune.com/2021/08/03/COVID-delta-variant-wave-uk-have-already-receded-us/.

9. Cocks T, "How South African Scientists Spotted the Omicron COVID Variant," Reuters, November 30, 2021, https://www.reuters.com/business/healthcare-pharmaceuticals/how-south-african-scientists-spotted-omicron-COVID-variant-2021-11-30/.

10. Kozlov M, "Omicron's Feeble Attack on the Lungs Could Make It Less Dangerous," *Nature* 601, no. 7892 (2022): 177, https://doi.org/10.1038/d41586-022-00007-8.

11. Harris JE, "COVID-19 Incidence and Hospitalization During the Delta Surge Were Inversely Related to Vaccination Coverage Among the Most Populous U.S. Counties," *Health Policy and Technology* 11, no. 2 (2022): 100583, https://doi.org/10.1016/j.hlpt.2021.100583.

12. Deol T, "Nearly 60% of Global Population to Be Infected with Omicron by March: IHME," Down to Earth, January 12, 2022, https://www.downtoearth.org.in/news/health/nearly-60-of-global-population-to-be-infected-with-omicron-by-march-ihme-81086.

13. Clarke KEN, Jones JM, Deng Y, et al., "Seroprevalence of Infection-Induced SARS-CoV-2 Antibodies—United States, September 2021–February 2022," *Morbidity and Mortality Weekly Report* 71, no. 17 (2022): 606–608, https://doi.org/10.15585/mmwr.mm7117e3.

14. CDC, "Nationwide Commercial Lab Pediatric Antibody Seroprevalence," September 2022, https://COVID.cdc.gov/COVID-data-tracker /#pediatric-seroprevalence.

15. Steenhuysen J, Roy M, "WHO Lays Out Plan to Emerge from Emergency Phase of Pandemic," Reuters, March 30, 2022, https://www .reuters.com/business/healthcare-pharmaceuticals/who-lays-out-plan -emerge-emergency-phase-pandemic-2022-03-30/; Pronczuk M, "The European Union Says the Emergency Phase of the Pandemic Is Over," *New York Times,* April 27, 2022, https://www.nytimes.com/2022/04/27 /world/european-union-COVID.html; Achenbach J, Pietsch B, "U.S. No Longer in 'Full-Blown' Pandemic Phase, Fauci Says," *Washington Post,* April 27, 2022, https://www.washingtonpost.com/health/2022/04/27 /pandemic-phase-over-fauci-COVID/.

16. European Centre for Disease Prevention and Control, "Transitioning Beyond the Acute Phase of the COVID-19 Pandemic," April 27, 2022, https://www.ecdc.europa.eu/sites/default/files/documents/Transitioning-beyond-the-acute-phase-of-the-COVID-19-pandemic_27April2022 .pdf; Massetti GM, Jackson BR, Brooks JT, et al., "Summary of Guidance for Minimizing the Impact of COVID-19 on Individual Persons, Communities, and Health Care Systems—United States, August 2022," *Morbidity and Mortality Weekly Report* 71, no. 33 (2022): 1057–1064, https://doi.org/10.15585/mmwr.mm7133e1.

17. Lazar K, "Prominent Doctor Faces Backlash amid 'Fight over the Heart of Public Health,'" *Boston Globe,* September 1, 2022, https://www .bostonglobe.com/2022/09/01/metro/prominent-doctor-faces-backlash -amid-fight-over-heart-public-health/; California State Legislature, "SB-1479: COVID-19 Testing in Schools: COVID-19 Testing Plans," October 2022, https://leginfo.legislature.ca.gov/faces/billNavClient .xhtml?bill_id=202120220SB1479.

18. Dupont SC, Galea S, "Science, Competing Values, and Trade-offs in Public Health—The Example of COVID-19 and Masking," *New England Journal of Medicine* 387, no. 10 (2022): 865–867, https://doi.org/10.1056 /NEJMp2207670.

19. Halperin DT, Hearst N, Hodgins S, et al., "Revisiting COVID-19 Policies: 10 Evidence-Based Recommendations for Where to Go from Here," *BMC Public Health* 21, no. 1 (2021): 2084, https://doi.org/10 .1186/s12889-021-12082-z.

20. Noble JA, "A Rational Roadmap to Future COVID Management," Smerconish, March 22, 2022, https://www.smerconish.com

/exclusive-content/a-rational-roadmap-to-future-COVID
-management/.

21. Gandhi M, "Overcaution Carries Its Own Danger to Children," *The Atlantic,* February 2021, https://www.theatlantic.com/ideas/archive
/2021/02/vaccines-are-banishing-any-debate-about-reopening
-schools/618155/; Hoeg TB, Henderson TO, Johnson D, Gandhi M,
"Our Next National Priority Should Be to Reopen All America's Schools
for Full Time In-Person Learning," *The Hill,* March 20, 2021, https://
thehill.com/opinion/healthcare/544142-our-next-national-priority
-should-be-to-reopen-all-americas-schools-for/; Madad S, Gandhi M,
Jha A, "These Are the Metrics That Will Tell Us When We Can Safely
Lift Restrictions," *Washington Post,* April 7, 2021, https://www
.washingtonpost.com/outlook/2021/04/07/COVID-vaccine-lift
-restrictions/; Hoeg TB, Gandhi M, Brown L, "Widespread Coronavirus
Surveillance Testing at Schools Is a Bad Idea," *Washington Post,* April 19,
2021, https://www.washingtonpost.com/outlook/2021/04/19/schools
-COVID-testing-cost/; Hoeg TB, Gandhi M, Johnson D, "We Must
Fully Reopen Schools This Fall. Here's How," *New York Times*, June 8,
2021, https://www.nytimes.com/2021/06/08/opinion/blueprint
-reopening-schools.html; Gandhi M, Noble J, "The Pandemic's Toll on
Teen Mental Health," *Wall Street Journal,* June 10, 2021, https://www
.wsj.com/articles/the-pandemics-toll-on-teen-mental-health-116233
44542; Gandhi, "We Won't Eradicate COVID. The Pandemic Will
Still End"; Vergales J, Gandhi M, "School Quarantines Keep Too Many
Kids at Home—with Barely Any Effect on COVID," *Washington Post,*
October 5, 2021, https://www.washingtonpost.com/outlook/2021/10/05
/quarantine-COVID-schools-modified-test/; Gandhi M, Bienen L, "Why
Hospitalizations Are Now a Better Indicator of COVID's Impact," *New
York Times,* December 11, 2021, https://www.nytimes.com/2021/12/11
/opinion/why-hospitalizations-are-now-a-better-indicator-of-COVIDs
-impact.html; Gandhi M, Noble J, "We Can't Just Impose Restrictions
Whenever COVID 19 Surges. Here's a Better Plan for 2022," *Time,*
December 22, 2021, https://time.com/6131104/rethinking-COVID-19
-restrictions-2022/.

22. Wilson N, Mansoor OD, Boyd MJ, et al., "We Should Not Dismiss the
Possibility of Eradicating COVID-19: Comparisons with Smallpox and
Polio," *BMJ Global Health* 6, no. 8 (2021): e006810, https://doi.org/10
.1136/bmjgh-2021-006810.

23. Burn-Murdoch J, Barnes O, "Vaccines and Omicron Mean COVID
Now Less Deadly Than Flu in England," *Financial Times,* March 9, 2022,

https://www.ft.com/content/e26c93a0-90e7-4dec-a796-3e25e94
bc59b; Thomas N, Smout A, "'Freedom Day' or 'Anxiety Day'? England
to End COVID-19 Curbs," Reuters, July 15, 2021, https://www.reuters
.com/world/uk/freedom-day-or-anxiety-day-england-end-COVID-19
-curbs-2021-07-15/.

24. LaFraniere S, "'Very Harmful' Lack of Data Blunts U.S. Response to
Outbreaks," *New York Times,* September 20, 2022, https://www.nytimes
.com/2022/09/20/us/politics/COVID-data-outbreaks.html; Mandavilli
A, "The C.D.C. Isn't Publishing Large Portions of the COVID Data It
Collects," *New York Times,* February 20, 2022, https://www.nytimes
.com/2022/02/20/health/COVID-cdc-data.html.

25. Daignault M, Gandhi M, "Omicron, Delta, and the Need for More
Accurate Hospitalization Data," Smerconish, January 6, 2022, https://
www.smerconish.com/exclusive-content/omicron-delta-and-the-need
-for-more-accurate-hospitalization-data/.

26. Allan-Blitz L, Klausner JD, "Mandatory Hospital Screenings Fuel
Inaccurate COVID Death Counts," *The Hill,* August 31, 2022, https://
thehill.com/opinion/healthcare/3622402-mandatory-hospital-screenings
-fuel-inaccurate-COVID-death-counts/.

27. Banco E, "Biden Officials Trying to Recalculate U.S. COVID-19
Hospitalizations," *Politico,* February 7, 2022, https://www.politico.com
/news/2022/02/07/biden-COVID-hospitalization-data-recalculate
-00006341.

28. Doron S, "An Epidemiologist's Advice for Living with COVID,"
CommonWealth, October 2022, https://commonwealthmagazine.org
/health/an-epidemiologists-advice-for-living-with-COVID/.

29. Moffa MA, Shively NR, Carr DR, et al., "Description of Hospitalizations
Due to the Severe Acute Respiratory Syndrome Coronavirus 2 Omicron
Variant Based on Vaccination Status," *Open Forum Infectious Diseases*
9, no. 9 (2022): ofac438, https://doi.org/10.1093/ofid/ofac438; UK
Department of Health and Social Care, "Regular Asymptomatic Testing
Paused in Additional Settings," August 2022, https://www.gov.uk
/government/news/regular-asymptomatic-testing-paused-in
-additional-settings; CDC, "Interim Infection Prevention and Control
Recommendations for Healthcare Personnel During the Coronavirus
Disease 2019 (COVID-19) Pandemic," September 2022, https://www
.cdc.gov/coronavirus/2019-ncov/hcp/infection-control-recommendations
.html; SHEA, "Pre-Procedure and Pre-Admission COVID-19 Testing
No Longer Recommended for Asymptomatic Patients," December 21,
2022, https://shea-online.org/pre-procedure-and-pre-admission

-covid-19-testing-no-longer-recommended-for-asymptomatic
-patients/.

30. Tenforde MW, Self WH, Gaglani M, et al., "Effectiveness of mRNA
     Vaccination in Preventing COVID-19–Associated Invasive Mechanical
     Ventilation and Death—United States, March 2021–January 2022,"
     Morbidity and Mortality Weekly Report 71, no. 12 (2022): 459–465,
     https://doi.org/10.15585/mmwr.mm7112e1; Wherry EJ, et al., "T Cell
     Immunity to COVID-19 Vaccines," *Science* 377, no. 6608 (August 18,
     2022): 821–822, https://www.science.org/doi/10.1126/science.add
     2897.

31. Turner JS, O'Halloran JA, Kalaidina E, et al., "SARS-CoV-2 mRNA
     Vaccines Induce Persistent Human Germinal Centre Responses," *Nature*
     596, no. 7870 (2021): 109–113, https://doi.org/10.1038/s41586-021
     -03738-2; Goel RR, Painter MM, Apostolidis SA, et al., "mRNA
     Vaccines Induce Durable Immune Memory to SARS-CoV-2 and Variants
     of Concern," *Science* 374, no. 6572 (2021): abm0829, https://doi.org
     /10.1126/science.abm0829; Lyski ZL, et al., "Severe Acute Respiratory
     Syndrome Coronavirus 2 (SARS-CoV-2)–Specific Memory B Cells from
     Individuals with Diverse Disease Severities Recognize SARS-CoV-2
     Variants of Concern," *Journal of Infectious Diseases* (March 15, 2022):
     947–956, https://doi.org/10.1093/infdis/jiab585; Gandhi M, "Don't Panic
     over Waning Antibodies. Here's Why," Leaps, September 2, 2021, https://
     leaps.org/how-long-do-COVID-antibodies-last/; Gandhi M, "How
     Cellular Immunity Works in Reference to COVID-19, Vaccines, and
     Boosters," *Medscape,* October 28, 2022, https://www.med
     scape.com/viewarticle/983095.

32. Lyski et al., "Severe Acute Respiratory Syndrome Coronavirus 2 (SARS-
     CoV-2)–Specific Memory B Cells from Individuals with Diverse Disease
     Severities Recognize SARS-CoV-2 Variants of Concern."

33. Yu X, Tsibane T, McGraw PA, et al., "Neutralizing Antibodies Derived
     from the B Cells of 1918 Influenza Pandemic Survivors," *Nature* 455, no.
     7212 (2008): 532–536, https://doi.org/10.1038/nature07231.

34. Wherry et al., "T Cell immunity to COVID-19 Vaccines."

35. Dan JM, Mateus J, Kato Y, et al., "Immunological Memory to SARS-
     CoV-2 Assessed for up to 8 Months After Infection," *Science* 371, no.
     6529 (2021): eabf4063, https://doi.org/10.1126/science.abf4063.

36. Le Bert N, Tan AT, Kunasegaran K, et al., "SARS-CoV-2-Specific T Cell
     Immunity in Cases of COVID-19 and SARS, and Uninfected Controls,"
     Nature 584, no. 7821 (2020): 457–462, https://doi.org/10.1038/s41586
     -020-2550-z.

37. Tenforde et al., "Effectiveness of mRNA Vaccination in Preventing COVID-19–Associated Invasive Mechanical Ventilation and Death—United States, March 2021–January 2022."

38. McCluskey PD, "Why This Wave of COVID Hospitalizations in Mass. Is Different," WBUR, June 1, 2022, https://www.wbur.org/news/2022/06/01/COVID-hospitals-massachusetts-different-wave.

39. Vu C, Kawaguchi ES, Torres CH, et al., "A More Accurate Measurement of COVID-19 Hospitalizations," *medRxiv,* June 2022, https://doi.org/10.1101/2022.06.03.22275891.

40. Gains J, "WHO: Global COVID Deaths Drop 90 Percent Since February," *The Hill,* November 10, 2022, https://thehill.com/policy/healthcare/3729252-who-global-COVID-deaths-drop-90-percent-since-february/.

41. Richardson JR, Götz R, Mayr V, et al., "SARS-CoV2 Wild Type and Mutant Specific Humoral and T Cell Immunity Is Superior After Vaccination Than After Natural Infection," *PLOS ONE* 17, no. 4 (2022): e0266701, https://doi.org/10.1371/journal.pone.0266701.

42. US FDA, "Coronavirus (COVID-19) Update: FDA Authorizes Moderna, Pfizer-BioNTech Bivalent COVID-19 Vaccines for Use as a Booster Dose," press release, August 31, 2022, https://www.fda.gov/news-events/press-announcements/coronavirus-COVID-19-update-fda-authorizes-moderna-pfizer-biontech-bivalent-COVID-19-vaccines-use.

43. Altarawneh HN, Chemaitelly H, Ayoub HH, et al., "Effects of Previous Infection and Vaccination on Symptomatic Omicron Infections," *New England Journal of Medicine* 387, no. 1 (2022): 21–34, https://doi.org/10.1056/NEJMoa2203965.

44. Daignault M, Gandhi M, "Immune Cells Mean Omicron Won't Swamp Hospitals in Vaccinated Areas," *Washington Post,* December 23, 2021, https://www.washingtonpost.com/outlook/2021/12/23/immune-cells-COVID-hospitals/; Gandhi M, "BA.4 and BA.5 Subvariants Are More Evasive of Antibodies, but Not of Cellular Immunity," *Medscape,* July 12, 2022, https://www.medscape.com/viewarticle/976945; Gandhi M, "How Cellular Immunity Works in Reference to COVID-19, Vaccines, and Boosters," *Medscape,* October 28, 2022, https://www.medscape.com/viewarticle/983095.

45. Jung MK, Jeong SD, Noh JY, et al., "BNT162b2-Induced Memory T Cells Respond to the Omicron Variant with Preserved Polyfunctionality," *Nature Microbiology* 7, no. 6 (2022): 909–917, https://doi.org/10.1038/s41564-022-01123-x; Wherry et al., "T Cell Immunity to COVID-19 Vaccines."

46. Koutsakos M, Lee WS, Reynaldi A, et al., "The Magnitude and Timing of Recalled Immunity After Breakthrough Infection Is Shaped by SARS-CoV-2 Variants," *Immunity* 55, no. 7 (2022): 1316–1326.e4, https://doi .org/10.1016/j.immuni.2022.05.018.

47. Goel RR, Painter MM, Apostolidis SA, et al., "mRNA Vaccines Induce Durable Immune Memory to SARS-CoV-2 and Variants of Concern," *Science* 374, no. 6572 (2021): abm0829, https://doi.org/10.1126/science .abm0829.

48. Lee H, "More Than 6 in 10 Elderly Koreans Fully Vaccinated, Boosted," *Korea Biomedical Review,* December 22, 2021, http://www.koreabiomed .com/news/articleView.html?idxno=12822.

49. Butt AA, Talisa VB, Shaikh OS, et al., "Relative Vaccine Effectiveness of a Severe Acute Respiratory Syndrome Coronavirus 2 Messenger RNA Vaccine Booster Dose Against the Omicron Variant," *Clinical Infectious Diseases* (2022): ciac328, https://doi.org/10.1093/cid/ciac328.

50. Gazit S, Saciuk Y, Perez G, Peretz A, et al., "Short Term, Relative Effectiveness of Four Doses Versus Three Doses of BNT162b2 Vaccine in People Aged 60 Years and Older in Israel: Retrospective, Test Negative, Case-Control Study," *BMJ* 377 (2022): e071113, https://doi.org/10.1136 /bmj-2022-071113; Minervina AA, Pogorelyy MV, Kirk AM, et al., "SARS-CoV-2 Antigen Exposure History Shapes Phenotypes and Specificity of Memory CD8+ T Cells," *Nature Immunology* 23, no. 5 (2022): 781–790, https://doi.org/10.1038/s41590-022-01184-4; Muecksch F, Wang Z, Cho A, et al., "Increased Memory B Cell Potency and Breadth After a SARS-CoV-2 mRNA Boost," *Nature* 607, no. 7917 (2022): 128–134, https://doi.org/10.1038/s41586-022-04 778-y.

51. Doron S, Gandhi M, "New Boosters Are Here! Who Should Receive Them and When?," *Lancet Infectious Diseases,* October 27, 2022, https:// doi.org/10.1016/S1473-3099(22)00688-0.

52. Crotty S, "Hybrid Immunity," *Science* 372, no. 6549 (2021): 1392–1393, https://doi.org/10.1126/science.abj2258; Gandhi M, "Immunity Against the Omicron Variant from Vaccination, Recovery, or Both," *Clinical Infectious Diseases* 75, no. 1 (2022): e672–e674, https://doi.org/10.1093 /cid/ciac172; Altarawneh HN, et al., "Effects of Previous Infection and Vaccination on Symptomatic Omicron Infections," *New England Journal of Medicine* 387 (July 7, 2022): 21–34, https://www.nejm.org/doi/10 .1056/NEJMoa2203965.

53. Lim JME, Tan AT, Le Bert N, et al., "SARS-CoV-2 Breakthrough Infection in Vaccinees Induces Virus-Specific Nasal-Resident CD8+ and

CD4+ T Cells of Broad Specificity," *Journal of Experimental Medicine* 219, no. 10 (2022): e20220780, https://doi.org/10.1084/jem.20220780.

54. "Booster After Infection Adds Little Extra Benefit vs Omicron," MDLinx, May 5, 2022, https://www.mdlinx.com/news/booster-after-infection-adds-little-extra-benefit-vs-omicron/3bPrgMMdBFWmkes7KbOfGm; Lim et al., "SARS-CoV-2 Breakthrough Infection in Vaccinees Induces Virus-Specific Nasal-Resident CD8+ and CD4+ T Cells of Broad Specificity"; Doron and Gandhi, "New Boosters Are Here"; Agrawal U, Bedston S, McCowan C, et al., "Severe COVID-19 Outcomes After Full Vaccination of Primary Schedule and Initial Boosters: Pooled Analysis of National Prospective Cohort Studies of 30 Million Individuals in England, Northern Ireland, Scotland, and Wales," *Lancet* 400, no. 10360 (2022): 1305–1320, doi: 10.1016/S0140-6736(22)01656-7.

55. Goldberg Y, Mandel M, Bar-On YM, et al., "Protection and Waning of Natural and Hybrid Immunity to SARS-CoV-2," *New England Journal of Medicine* 386, no. 23 (2022): 2201–2212, https://doi.org/10.1056/NEJ Moa2118946.

56. "The Power of mRNA," Moderna, https://www.modernatx.com/power-of-mrna/science-of-mrna?tc=ps_zw3e5fv&cc=1001.

57. Xiang D, Lehmann LS, "Confronting the Misinformation Pandemic," *Health Policy and Technology* 10, no. 3 (2021): 100520, https://doi.org/10.1016/j.hlpt.2021.100520.

58. WHO, "Infodemic," 2022, https://www.who.int/health-topics/infodemic.

59. CDC, "Percent of the Population 5 Years of Age and Older with at Least One Dose Reported to CDC by Jurisdictions and Select Federal Entities," September 2022, https://COVID.cdc.gov/COVID-data-tracker/#vaccinations_vacc-people-onedose-pop-5yr; Holder J, "Tracking Coronavirus Vaccinations Around the World," *New York Times,* January 2021, https://www.nytimes.com/interactive/2021/world/COVID-vaccinations-tracker.html.

60. Gandhi M, Daignault M, "We Need to Clarify the Goal of Our COVID Booster Strategy," *MedPage Today,* March 30, 2022, https://www.medpagetoday.com/opinion/second-opinions/97948.

61. Geddes L, "What Is the Novavax Vaccine, and Why Does the World Need Another Type of COVID-19 Vaccine?," GAVI, February 14, 2022, https://www.gavi.org/vaccineswork/what-novavax-vaccine-and-why-does-world-need-another-type-COVID-19-vaccine; Dolgin E, "How Protein-Based COVID Vaccines Could Change the Pandemic," *Nature* 599, no. 7885 (2021): 359–360, https://doi.org/10.1038/d41586-021-03025-0.

62. US FDA, "Vaccines and Related Biological Products Advisory Committee June 7, 2022 Meeting Announcement," June 7, 2022, https:// www.fda.gov/advisory-committees/advisory-committee-calendar /vaccines-and-related-biological-products-advisory-committee-june-7 -2022-meeting-announcement; CDC, "CDC Allows Novavax Monovalent COVID-19 Boosters for Adults Ages 18 and Older," October 19, 2022, https://www.cdc.gov/media/releases/2022/s1019-novavax .html; Gandhi M, "Novavax and Covaxin: What You Need to Know," *Medscape,* June 6, 2022, https://www.medscape.com/viewarticle /975110.

63. Keech C, Albert G, Cho I, et al., "Phase 1–2 Trial of a SARS-CoV-2 Recombinant Spike Protein Nanoparticle Vaccine," *New England Journal of Medicine* 383, no. 24 (2020): 2320–2332, https://doi.org/10.1056 /NEJMoa2026920.

64. Keech et al., "Phase 1–2 Trial of a SARS-CoV-2 Recombinant Spike Protein Nanoparticle Vaccine."

65. CDC, "Adjuvants and Vaccines," September 2022, https://www.cdc.gov /vaccinesafety/concerns/adjuvants.html.

66. Ocugen, "Ocugen Secures Manufacturing Partnership for US Production of COVID-19 Vaccine Candidate, COVAXIN," press release, June 15, 2021, https://ir.ocugen.com/news-releases/news-release-details /ocugen-secures-manufacturing-partnership-us-production-COVID-19/; Gandhi, "Novavax and Covaxin: What You Need to Know."

67. Taylor A, "WHO Backs Extra Jab for Chinese-Made Vaccines, Despite Resistance to Coronavirus Boosters over Supply Strain," *Washington Post,* October 12, 2021, https://www.washingtonpost.com/world/2021/10/12 /sinovac-sinopharm-third-dose/.

68. NIH, "Adjuvant Developed with NIH Funding Enhances Efficacy of India's COVID 19 Vaccine," press release, June 29, 2021, https://www .nih.gov/news-events/news-releases/adjuvant-developed-nih-funding -enhances-efficacy-indias-COVID-19-vaccine.

69. Edara VV, Patel M, Suthar MS, "Covaxin (BBV152) Vaccine Neutralizes SARS-CoV-2 Delta and Omicron Variants," *medRxiv,* January 2022, https://doi.org/10.1101/2022.01.24.22269189; Vikkurthi R, et al., "Inactivated Whole-Virion Vaccine BBV152/Covaxin Elicits Robust Cellular Immune Memory to SARS-CoV-2 and Variants of Concern," *Nature Microbiology* 7 (June 9, 2022): 974–985, https://www.nature.com /articles/s41564-022-01161-5.

70. Ocugen, "Ocugen Provides an Update on Its COVAXIN Pediatric (2–18) Emergency Use Authorization (EUA) Request," press release, March 4,

2022, https://ir.ocugen.com/news-releases/news-release-details/ocugen
-provides-update-its-covaxintm-pediatric-2-18-emergency/.

71. Ocugen, "A Phase 2/3, Observer-Blind, Immuno-Bridging, and
Broadening Study of a Whole, Inactivated Severe Acute Respiratory
Syndrome Coronavirus (SARS-CoV-2) Vaccine (BBV152) in Healthy
Adults (Clinical Trial Registration No. NCT05258669)," ClinicalTrials
.gov, last updated August 31, 2022, https://clinicaltrials.gov/ct2/show
/NCT05258669.

72. Hui KP, Ng KC, Ho JC, et al., "Replication of SARS-CoV-2 Omicron
BA.2 Variant in Ex Vivo Cultures of the Human Upper and Lower
Respiratory Tract," SSRN, May 2022, https://doi.org/10.2139/ssrn
.4123178.

73. Hammond J, Leister-Tebbe H, Gardner A, et al., "Oral Nirmatrelvir for
High-Risk, Nonhospitalized Adults with COVID-19," *New England
Journal of Medicine* 386, no. 15 (2022): 1397–1408, https://doi.org/10
.1056/NEJMoa2118542.

74. Arbel R, Wolff Sagy Y, Hoshen M, et al., "Nirmatrelvir Use and Severe
COVID-19 Outcomes During the Omicron Surge," *New England Journal
of Medicine* 387, no. 9 (2022): 790–798, https://doi.org/10.1056/NEJM
oa2204919.

75. Malden DE, Hong V, Lewin BJ, et al., "Hospitalization and Emergency
Department Encounters for COVID-19 After Paxlovid Treatment—
California, December 2021–May 2022," *Morbidity and Mortality Weekly
Report* 71, no. 25 (2022): 830–833, https://doi.org/10.15585/mmwr
.mm7125e2.

76. Arbel et al., "Nirmatrelvir Use and Severe COVID-19 Outcomes During
the Omicron Surge."

77. Bernal AJ et al., "Molnupiravir for Oral Treatment of Covid-19 in
Nonhospitalized Patients," *New England Journal of Medicine* 386 (2022):
509-520, https://www.nejm.org/doi/full/10.1056/NEJMoa2116044;
Johnson MG et al., "Molnupiravir for the Treatment of COVID-19
in Immunocompromised Participants: Efficacy, Safety, and Virology
Results from the Phase 3 Randomized, Placebo-Controlled MOVe-
OUT Trial," *Infection* (2023), https://link.springer.com/article/10.1007/
s15010-022-01959-9.

78. Butler CB et al., "Molnupiravir Plus Usual Care versus Usual Care Alone
as Early Treatment for Adults with COVID-19 at Increased Risk of
Adverse Outcomes (PANORAMIC): An Open-Label, Platform-Adaptive
Randomized Controlled Trial," *Lancet* (December 2022), https://doi
.org/10.1016/S0140-6736(22)02597-1.

79. U.S. Food & Drug Administration, "FDA Updates on Bebtelovimab," November 30, 2022, https://www.fda.gov/drugs/drug-safety-and -availability/fda-updates-bebtelovimab; U.S. Food & Drug Administration, "FDA Announces Bebtelovimab Is Not Currently Authorized in Any US Region," November 30, 2022, https://www.fda .gov/drugs/drug-safety-and-availability/fda-announces-bebtelovimab -not-currently-authorized-any-us-region.

80. Gandhi M, "COVID-19 Vaccines Work Better Than Expected," *Medscape,* May 27, 2022, https://www.medscape.com/viewarticle /974363.

81. Haidar G, Agha M, Bilderback A, et al., "Prospective Evaluation of Coronavirus Disease 2019 (COVID-19) Vaccine Responses Across a Broad Spectrum of Immunocompromising Conditions: The COVID-19 Vaccination in the Immunocompromised Study (COVICS)," *Clinical Infectious Diseases* 75, no. 1 (2022): e630–e644, https://doi.org/10.1093 /cid/ciac103.

82. Waldhorn I, Holland R, Goshen-Lago T, et al., "Long-Term Immunogenicity of BNT162b2 Vaccine in Patients with Solid Tumors," *JAMA Oncology* 8, no. 6 (2022): 940–941, https://doi.org/10.1001 /jamaoncol.2022.1467.

83. CDC, "COVID-19 Vaccines for People Who Are Moderately or Severely Immunocompromised," October 2022, https://www.cdc.gov/corona virus/2019-ncov/vaccines/recommendations/immuno.html.

84. AstraZeneca, "Evusheld Long-Acting Antibody Combination Retains Neutralising Activity Against Omicron Variants BA.4 and BA.5, According to New Study from University of Oxford," press release, May 25, 2022, https://www.astrazeneca.com/media-centre/medical -releases/evusheld-long-acting-antibody-combination-retains -neutralising-activity-omicron-variants-ba4-ba5-according-new-study -university-oxford.html; US FDA, "FDA Releases Important Information About Risk of COVID-19 Due to Certain Variants Not Neutralized by Evusheld," press release, October 3, 2022, https://www .fda.gov/drugs/drug-safety-and-availability/fda-releases-important -information-about-risk-COVID-19-due-certain-variants-not-neutralized -evusheld.

85. NIH, "The COVID-19 Treatment Guidelines Panel's Statement on Omicron Subvariants, Pre-Exposure Prophylaxis, and Therapeutic Management of Nonhospitalized Patients with COVID-19," November 10, 2022, https://www.COVID19treatmentguidelines.nih.gov/therapies /statement-on-omicron-subvariants/.

86. Ujifusa A, "How One Governor's Race Has Channeled National and Local Anger over Schools," *Education Week,* October 27, 2021, https://www.edweek.org/policy-politics/how-one-governors-race-has-channeled-national-and-local-anger-over-schools/2021/10.

87. Omer SB, "Vaccine Disruptions and Mistrust Are Ramping Up Measles Risk," *Los Angeles Times,* June 12, 2022, https://www.latimes.com/opinion/story/2022-06-12/vaccines-kids-measles-outbreaks; Doron S, Gandhi M, "Time to Come Clean about COVID-19: Bring Back 'May' versus 'Should' Language to Restore Trust," *CommonWealth,* November 26, 2022, https://commonwealthmagazine.org/health/time-to-come-clean-about-covid-19.

88. Leuchter RK, Jackson NJ, Mafi JN, et al., "Association Between COVID-19 Vaccination and Influenza Vaccination Rates," *New England Journal of Medicine* 386, no. 26 (2022): 2531–2532, https://www.nejm.org/doi/full/10.1056/NEJMc2204560.

89. Guilfoil K, "Less Than 60% of Kids Are Vaccinated Against Polio in Some NYC Neighborhoods," ABC News, August 19, 2022, https://abcnews.go.com/Health/60-kids-vaccinated-polio-nyc-neighborhoods/story?id=88550152.

90. Reardon S, "First U.S. Polio Case in Nearly a Decade Highlights the Importance of Vaccination," *Scientific American,* August 19, 2022, https://www.scientificamerican.com/article/first-u-s-polio-case-in-nearly-a-decade-highlights-the-importance-of-vaccination/; Bendix A, "New York Declared a State of Emergency over Polio," NBC News, September 9, 2022, https://www.nbcnews.com/health/health-news/new-york-polio-state-of-emergency-rcna47054; Gandhi M, "Polio Making a Comeback in the US Owing to Declining Vaccination Rates," *Medscape,* September 19, 2022, https://www.medscape.com/viewarticle/980857.

91. Maricopa County Department of Public Health, "Three Measles Cases Confirmed in Maricopa County," September 1, 2022, https://www.maricopa.gov/CivicAlerts.aspx?AID=2567; Breen K, "Several Children Hospitalized in Growing Measles Outbreak Affecting 7 Ohio Daycares," CBS News, November 16, 2022, https://www.cbsnews.com/news/children-hospitalized-measles-outbreak-ohio-daycares-columbus/.

92. Hostetter M, Klein S, "Understanding and Ameliorating Medical Mistrust Among Black Americans," Commonwealth Fund, January 14, 2021, https://doi.org/10.26099/9GRT-2B21.

93. UNICEF, "COVID-19: Scale of Education Loss 'Nearly Insurmountable,' Warns UNICEF," press release, January 23, 2022,

https://www.unicef.org/press-releases/COVID19-scale-education-loss
-nearly-insurmountable-warns-unicef.

CHAPTER 4: RESOURCES BEFORE RESTRICTIONS,
AND THE DUTY OF PUBLIC HEALTH

1. Galvani AP, Parpia AS, Pandey A, Sah P, Colón K, Friedman G, Campbell T, Kahn JG, Singer BH, Fitzpatrick MC, "Universal Healthcare as Pandemic Preparedness: The Lives and Costs That Could Have Been Saved During the COVID-19 Pandemic," *Proceedings of the National Academy of Sciences* 119, no. 25 (2022): e2200536119, https://www.pnas.org/doi/full/10.1073/pnas.2200536119.

2. Gandhi M, Prasad V, Baral S, "What Does Public Health Really Mean? Lessons from COVID-19," *BMJ Opinion* (blog), July 26, 2021, https://blogs.bmj.com/bmj/2021/07/26/what-does-public-health-really-mean-lessons-from-COVID-19/.

3. Broadbent A, Walker D, Chalkidou K, Sullivan R, Glassman A, "Lockdown Is Not Egalitarian: The Costs Fall on the Global Poor," *Lancet* 396, no. 10243 (2020): 21–22, https://www.sciencedirect.com/science/article/pii/S0140673620314227.

4. Blake KD, Blendon RJ, Viswanath K, "Employment and Compliance with Pandemic Influenza Mitigation Recommendations," *Emerging Infectious Diseases* 16, no. 2 (2010): 212–218, https://wwwnc.cdc.gov/eid/article/16/2/09-0638_article.

5. Gettleman J, Schultz K, "Modi Orders 3-Week Total Lockdown for All 1.3 Billion Indians," *New York Times,* March 24, 2020, https://www.nytimes.com/2020/03/24/world/asia/india-coronavirus-lockdown.html; Pandey V, "Coronavirus Lockdown: The Indian Migrants Dying to Get Home," BBC, May 20, 2020, https://www.bbc.com/news/world-asia-india-52672764.

6. Ahmed T, Roberton T, Vergeer P, et al., "Healthcare Utilization and Maternal and Child Mortality During the COVID-19 Pandemic in 18 Low- and Middle-Income Countries: An Interrupted Time-Series Analysis with Mathematical Modeling of Administrative Data," *PLOS Medicine* 19, no. 8 (2022): e1004070, https://journals.plos.org/plosmedicine/article?id=10.1371/journal.pmed.1004070.

7. Yoo KJ, Millward J, Bishai DM, et al., "Excess Under-Five Mortality Due to COVID-19 Related Economic Downturn," *Investing in Health* (World Bank blog), April 15, 2022, https://blogs.worldbank.org/health

/excess-under-five-mortality-due-COVID-19-related-economic
-downturn.

8. Massetti GM, Jackson BR, Brooks JT, et al., "Summary of Guidance
for Minimizing the Impact of COVID-19 on Individual Persons,
Communities, and Health Care Systems—United States, August 2022,"
Morbidity and Mortality Weekly Report 71, no. 33 (2022): 1057–1064,
http://dx.doi.org/10.15585/mmwr.mm7133e1; Leonhardt D, "Our Latest
COVID Poll," *New York Times,* August 31, 2022, https://www.nytimes
.com/2022/08/31/briefing/COVID-poll-liberal-anxiety.html.

9. Gandhi M, Carroll A, "The New Phase of the Pandemic Is COVID
Exhaustion," *New York Times,* March 9, 2022, https://www.nytimes
.com/2022/03/09/opinion/COVID-exhaustion-the-argument.html.

10. Marcus J, "The Danger of Assuming That Family Time Is Dispensable,"
The Atlantic, December 2020, https://www.theatlantic.com/ideas
/archive/2020/12/tis-the-season-for-shame-and-judgment/617335/.

11. Barocas J, Gandhi M, "Harm Reduction Principles Can Help Us Restore
Trust in Public Health Messaging on COVID-19," *BMJ Opinion* (blog),
December 15, 2020, https://blogs.bmj.com/bmj/2020/12/15/harm
-reduction-principles-can-help-us-restore-trust-in-public-health
-messaging-on-COVID-19/.

12. "Ipsos Issues Index: September 2022," Ipsos, https://www.ipsos.com/en
-uk/ipsos-issues-index-september-2022.

13. Blum D, "Another COVID Wave Could Be Coming. Here's How to
Make Your Holiday Plans," *New York Times,* October 15, 2022, https://
www.nytimes.com/2022/10/15/well/COVID-holiday-plans.html.

14. National Center for Education Statistics, US Department of Education,
"Reading and Mathematics Scores Decline During COVID-19
Pandemic," NAEP, 2020 and 2022 Long-Term Trend (LTT) Reading
and Mathematics Assessments, https://www.nationsreportcard.gov
/highlights/ltt/2022/; Hallin AE, Danielsson H, Nordström T, Fälth
L, "No Learning Loss in Sweden During the Pandemic: Evidence
from Primary School Reading Assessments," *International Journal of
Educational Research* 114 (2022): 102011, doi:10.1016/j.ijer.2022
.102011.

15. Green E, "The Liberals Who Can't Quit Lockdown," *The Atlantic,* May
2021, https://www.theatlantic.com/politics/archive/2021/05/liberals
-COVID-19-science-denial-lockdown/618780/.

16. UNAIDS, "In Danger: UNAIDS Global AIDS Update 2022," July 27,
2022, https://www.unaids.org/en/resources/documents/2022/in-danger
-global-aids-update.

17. Spinelli MA, Hickey MD, Glidden DV, et al., "Viral Suppression Rates in a Safety-Net HIV Clinic in San Francisco Destabilized During COVID-19," *AIDS* 34, no. 15 (2022): 2328–2331, doi:10.1097/QAD .0000000000002677.

18. Spinelli MA, Le Tourneau N, Glidden DV, et al., "Impact of Multicomponent Support Strategies on Human Immunodeficiency Virus Virologic Suppression Rates During Coronavirus Disease 2019: An Interrupted Time Series Analysis," *Clinical Infectious Diseases* 75, no. 1 (2022): e947–e954, doi:10.1093/cid/ciac179.

19. Gandhi M, "Monkeypox and COVID: Public Health Has to Increase Trust," *Medscape,* June 28, 2022, https://www.medscape.com/view article/976081.

20. Marcus, "The Danger of Assuming That Family Time Is Dispensable."

21. Jemmott JB, Jemmott LS, Fong GT, "Abstinence and Safer Sex HIV Risk-Reduction Interventions for African American Adolescents: A Randomized Controlled Trial," *Journal of the American Medical Association* 279, no. 19 (1998): 1529–1536, doi:10.1001/jama.279.19 .1529.

22. Chinazzi M, Davis JT, Ajelli M, et al., "The Effect of Travel Restrictions on the Spread of the 2019 Novel Coronavirus (COVID-19) Outbreak," *Science* 368, no. 6489 (2020): 395–400, doi:10.1126/science .aba9757.

23. Hernandez J, "African Leaders Condemn Travel Restrictions as Omicron Variant Spreads Globally," NPR, November 30, 2021, https://www.npr .org/sections/goatsandsoda/2021/11/30/1059780197/african-leaders -condemn-travel-restrictions-as-omicron-variant-spreads-globally.

24. Tan ST, Kwan AT, Rodríguez-Barraquer I, Singer BJ, Park HJ, Lewnard JA, Sears D, Lo NC, "Infectiousness of SARS-CoV-2 Breakthrough Infections and Reinfections During the Omicron Wave," *medRxiv,* August 8, 2022, https://doi.org/10.1101/2022.08.08.22278547.

25. US Department of Homeland Security, "DHS Extends COVID-19 Vaccination Requirements for Non-U.S. Travelers Entering the United States via Land Ports of Entry and Ferry Terminals," press release, April 21, 2022, https://www.dhs.gov/news/2022/04/21/dhs-extends-COVID -19-vaccination-requirements-non-us-travelers-entering-united.

26. Mineo L, "Remote Learning Likely Widened Racial, Economic Achievement Gap," *Harvard Gazette,* May 2022, https://news.harvard .edu/gazette/story/2022/05/remote-learning-likely-widened-racial -economic-achievement-gap/.

CHAPTER 5: SCHOOL CLOSURES AND COVID-19

1. Klaiman T, Kraemer JD, Stoto MA, "Variability in School Closure Decisions in Response to 2009 H1N1: A Qualitative Systems Improvement Analysis," *BMC Public Health* 11 (2011): 73, https://doi.org/10.1186/1471-2458-11-73; Cauchemez S, Ferguson NM, Wachtel C, Tegnell A, Saour G, Duncan B, Nicoll A, "Closure of Schools During an Influenza Pandemic," *Lancet Infectious Diseases* 9, no. 8 (2009): 473–481, https://doi.org/10.1016/S1473-3099(09)70176-8; Cauchemez S, Van Kerkhove MD, Archer BN, Cetron M, Cowling BJ, Grove P, Hunt D, et al., "School Closures During the 2009 Influenza Pandemic: National and Local Experiences," *BMC Infectious Diseases* 14 (2014): art. 207, https://doi.org/10.1186/1471-2334-14-207.

2. Stern AM, Reilly MB, Cetron MS, Markel H, "'Better Off in School': School Medical Inspection as a Public Health Strategy During the 1918–1919 Influenza Pandemic in the United States," *Public Health Reports* 25, supp. 3 (2010): 63–70, https://doi.org/10.1177/00333549101250S309.

3. "Boston, Massachusetts, and the 1918–1919 Influenza Epidemic," *The American Influenza Epidemic of 1918–1919: A Digital Encyclopedia,* University of Michigan Center for the History of Medicine and Michigan Publishing, accessed July 16, 2022, https://www.influenzaarchive.org/cities/city-boston.html; "Philadelphia, Pennsylvania, and the 1918–1919 Influenza Epidemic," *The American Influenza Epidemic of 1918–1919: A Digital Encyclopedia,* University of Michigan Center for the History of Medicine and Michigan Publishing, accessed July 16, 2022, https://www.influenzaarchive.org/cities/city-philadelphia.html; Aimone F, "The 1918 Influenza Epidemic in New York City: A Review of the Public Health Response," *Public Health Reports* 125, supp. 3 (2010): 71–79, https://doi.org/10.1177/00333549101250S310.

4. Markel H, Lipman HB, Navarro JA, Sloan A, Michalsen JR, Stern AM, Cetron MS, "Nonpharmaceutical Interventions Implemented by US Cities During the 1918–1919 Influenza Pandemic," *Journal of the American Medical Association* 298, no. 6 (2007): 644–654, https://doi.org/1001/jama.298.6.644.

5. Jayasundara K, Soobiah C, Thommes E, Tricco AC, Chit A, "Natural Attack Rate of Influenza in Unvaccinated Children and Adults: A Meta-Regression Analysis," *BMC Infectious Diseases* 14 (2014): art. 670, https://doi.org/10.1186/s12879-014-0670-5.

6. Rashid H, Ridda I, King C, Begun M, Tekin H, Wood JG, Booy R, "Evidence Compendium and Advice on Social Distancing and Other Related Measures for Response to an Influenza Pandemic," *Paediatric Respiratory Reviews* 16, no. 2 (2014): 119–126, https://doi.org/10.1016/j.prrv.2014.01.003.

7. Levinson M, Geller AC, Allen JG, "Health Equity, Schooling Hesitancy, and the Social Determinants of Learning," *Lancet Regional Health* 2 (2021): 100032, https://doi.org/10.1016/j.lana.2021.100032.

8. Levinson M, Markovits D, "The Biggest Disruption in the History of American Education," *The Atlantic,* June 23, 2022, https://www.theatlantic.com/ideas/archive/2022/06/COVID-learning-loss-remote-school/661360/.

9. UNESCO Institute of Statistics, "Global Monitoring of School Closures Caused by COVID-19," accessed July 17, 2022, https://COVID19.uis.unesco.org/global-monitoring-school-closures-COVID19/country-dashboard/.

10. Castagnoli R, Votto M, Licari A, Brambilla I, Bruno R, Perlini S, Rovida F, Baldanti F, Marseglia GL, "Severe Acute Respiratory Syndrome Coronavirus 2 (SARS-CoV-2) Infection in Children and Adolescents: A Systematic Review," *JAMA Pediatrics* 174, no. 9 (2020): 882–889, https://doi.org/10.1001/jamapediatrics.2020.1467.

11. Götzinger F, Santiago-García B, Noguera-Julián A, Lanaspa M, Lancella L, Calò Carducci FI, Gabrovska N, et al., "COVID-19 in Children and Adolescents in Europe: A Multinational, Multicentre Cohort Study," *Lancet Child and Adolescent Health* 4, no. 9 (2020): 653–661, https://doi.org/10.1016/S2352-4642(20)30177-2.

12. Smith C, Odd D, Harwood R, Ward J, Linney M, Clark M, Hargreaves D, et al., "Deaths in Children and Young People in England After SARS-CoV-2 Infection During the First Pandemic Year," *Nature Medicine* 28 (2021): 185–192, https://doi.org/10.1038/s41591-021-01578-1.

13. Bertran M, Amin-Chowdhury Z, Davies H, et al., "COVID-19 Deaths in Children and Young People: Active Prospective National Surveillance, March 2020 to December 2021, England," *PLOS Medicine,* November 8, 2022, https://journals.plos.org/plosmedicine/article?id=10.1371/journal.pmed.1004118.

14. Chappell H, Patel R, Driessens C, Tarr AW, Irving WL, Tighe PJ, Jackson HJ, et al., "Immunocompromised Children and Young People Are at No Increased Risk of Severe COVID-19," *Journal of Infection* 84, no. 1 (2021): 31–39, https://doi.org/10.1016/j.jinf.2021.11.005.

15. Payne AB, Gilani Z, Godfred-Cato S, et al., "Incidence of Multisystem Inflammatory Syndrome in Children Among US Persons Infected with SARS-CoV-2," *JAMA Network Open* 4, no. 6 (June 10, 2021): e2116420, doi:10.1001/jamanetworkopen.2021.16420; Cowen L, "US Survey Suggests Low Rates of Multisystem Inflammatory Syndrome in Children with COVID-19," *Medicine Matters,* June 29, 2021, https:// rheumatology.medicinematters.com/mis-c/COVID-19/multisystem -inflammatory-syndrome-rare-complication/19311344.

16. Son MBF, Friedman K, "COVID-19: Multisystem Inflammatory Syndrome in Children (MIS-C) Clinical Features, Evaluation, and Diagnosis," UpToDate, April 28, 2022, https://www.uptodate.com /contents/COVID-19-multisystem-inflammatory-syndrome-in -children-mis-c-clinical-features-evaluation-and-diagnosis#disclaimer Content.

17. "Health Department–Reported Cases of Multisystem Inflammatory Syndrome in Children (MIS-C) in the United States," CDC COVID Data Tracker, last updated October 3, 2022, https://COVID.cdc.gov /COVID-data-tracker/#mis-national-surveillance.

18. Molteni E, Sudre CH, Canas LS, Bhopal SS, Hughes RC, Antonelli M, Murray B, et al., "Illness Duration and Symptom Profile in Symptomatic UK School-Aged Children Tested for SARS-CoV-2," *Lancet Child and Adolescent Health* 5, no. 10 (2021): 708–718, https://doi.org/10.1016 /S2352-4642(21)00198-X.

19. Farhadian S, Doron S, "Controlled Studies Ease Worries of Widespread Long COVID in Kids," STAT, February 14, 2022, https://www.stat news.com/2022/02/14/controlled-studies-ease-worries-widespread -long-COVID-kids/.

20. Joy G, Artico J, Kurdi J, Seraphim A, Lau C, Thornton GD, Oliveira MF, et al., "Prospective Case-Control Study of Cardiovascular Abnormalities 6 Months Following Mild COVID-19 in Healthcare Workers," *JACC: Cardiovascular Imaging* 14, no. 11 (May 8, 2021): 2155–2166, https://doi .org/10.1016/j.jcmg.2021.04.011.

21. Chappell et al., "Immunocompromised Children and Young People Are at No Increased Risk of Severe COVID-19"; European Centre for Disease Prevention and Control, "COVID-19 in Children and the Role of School Settings in Transmission—Second Update," July 8, 2021, https://www.ecdc.europa.eu/sites/default/files/documents/COVID-19 -in-children-and-the-role-of-school-settings-in-transmission-second -update.pdf.

22. European Centre for Disease Prevention and Control, "COVID-19 in Children and the Role of School Settings in Transmission—Second Update."

23. Lamaz S and the SKIDS Investigation Team, "Children and COVID-19 in Schools," *Science,* November 4, 2021, https://www.science.org/doi/10.1126/science.abj2042.

24. Tönshoff B, Müller B, Elling R, Renk H, Meissner P, Hengel H, Garbade SF, "Prevalence of SARS-CoV-2 Infection in Children and Their Parents in Southwest Germany," *JAMA Pediatrics* 175, no. 6 (2021): 1–8, https://doi.org/10.1001/jamapediatrics.2021.0001.

25. Falk A, Benda A, Falk P, Steffen S, Wallace Z, Høeg TB, "COVID-19 Cases and Transmission in 17 K–12 Schools—Wood County, Wisconsin, August 31–November 29, 2020," *Morbidity and Mortality Weekly Report* 70, no. 4 (2021): 136–140, http://dx.doi.org/10.15585/mmwr.mm7004e3; Gillespie DL, Meyers LA, Lachmann M, Redd SC, Zenilman JM, "The Experience of 2 Independent Schools with In-Person Learning During the COVID-19 Pandemic," *Journal of School Health* 91, no. 5 (2021): 347–355, https://doi.org/10.1111/josh.13008; Schoeps A, Hoffmann D, Tamm C, Vollmer B, Haag S, Kaffenberger T, Ferguson-Beiser K, et al., "Surveillance of SARS-CoV-2 Transmission in Educational Institutions, August to December 2020, Germany," *Epidemiology and Infection* 149 (2021): 1–9, https://doi.org/10.1017/S0950268821002077; Sasser P, McGuine T, Haraldsdottir K, Biese K, Goodavish L, Stevens B, Watson AM, "Reported COVID-19 Incidence in Wisconsin High School Athletes in Fall 2020," *Journal of Athletic Training* 57, no. 1 (2021): 59–64, https://doi.org/10.4085/1062-6050-0185.21; Gold JAW, Gettings JR, Kimball A, Franklin R, Rivera G, Morris E, Scott C, et al., "Clusters of SARS-CoV-2 Infection Among Elementary School Educators and Students in One School District—Georgia, December 2020–January 2021," *Morbidity and Mortality Weekly Report* 70, no. 8 (2021): 289–292, http://dx.doi.org/10.15585/mmwr.mm7008e4; Hershow RB, Wu K, Lewis NM, Milne AT, Currie D, Smith AR, Lloyd S, et al., "Low SARS-CoV-2 Transmission in Elementary Schools—Salt Lake County, Utah, December 3, 2020–January 31, 2021," *Morbidity and Mortality Weekly Report* 70, no. 12 (2021): 442–448, http://dx.doi.org/10.15585/mmwr.mm7012e3; Zimmerman KO, Ibukunoluwa CA, Brookhart MA, Boutzoukas AE, McGann KA, Smith MJ, Panayotti GM, et al., "Incidence and Secondary Transmission of SARS-CoV-2 Infections in Schools," *Pediatrics* 147, no. 4 (2021): e2020048090, https://doi.org/10.1542/peds.2020-048090; Varma

JK., Thamkittikasem J, Whitteemore K, Alexander M, Stephens DH, Arslanian K, Bray J, Long TG, "COVID-19 Infections Among Students and Staff in New York City Public Schools," *Pediatrics* 147, no. 5 (2021): e2021050605, https://doi.org/10.1542/peds.2021-050605.

26. Gold et al., "Clusters of SARS-CoV-2 Infection Among Elementary School Educators and Students in One School District—Georgia, December 2020–January 2021"; Van den Berg P, Schechter-Perkins EM, Jack RS, Epshtein I, Nelson R, Oster E, Branch-Elliman W, "Effectiveness of 3 Versus 6 Ft of Physical Distancing for Controlling Spread of Coronavirus Disease 2019 Among Primary and Secondary Students and Staff: A Retrospective, Statewide Cohort Study," *Clinical Infectious Diseases* 73, no. 10 (2021): 1871–1878, https://doi.org/10.1093/cid/ciab230.

27. Falk et al., "COVID-19 Cases and Transmission in 17 K–12 Schools—Wood County, Wisconsin, August 31–November 29, 2020."

28. Falk et al., "COVID-19 Cases and Transmission in 17 K–12 Schools—Wood County, Wisconsin, August 31–November 29, 2020"; Honein MA, Barrios LC, Brooks JT, "Data and Policy to Guide Opening Schools Safely to Limit the Spread of SARS-CoV-2 Infection," *Journal of the American Medical Association* 325, no. 9 (2021): 823–824, https://doi.org/10.1001/jama.2021.0374; Hershow et al., "Low SARS-CoV-2 Transmission in Elementary Schools—Salt Lake County, Utah, December 3, 2020–January 31, 2021"; Varma et al., "COVID-19 Infections Among Students and Staff in New York City Public Schools."

29. CDC, "Nearly 80 Percent of Teachers, School Staff, and Childcare Workers Receive at Least One Shot of COVID-19 Vaccine," April 6, 2021, https://www.cdc.gov/media/releases/2021/s0406-teachers-staff-vaccine.html.

30. Tan ST, Kwan AT, Rodríguez-Barraquer I, Singer BJ, Park HJ, Lewnard JA, Sears D, Lo NC, "Infectiousness of SARS-CoV-2 Breakthrough Infections and Reinfections During the Omicron Wave," *medRxiv*, October 20, 2022, https://doi.org/10.1101/2022.08.08.22278547; Milman O, Yelin I, Aharony N, Katz R, Herzel E, Ben-Tov A, Kuint J, et al., "Community-Level Evidence for SARS-CoV-2 Vaccine Protection of Unvaccinated Individuals," *Nature Medicine* 27 (2021): 1367–1369, https://doi.org/10.1038/s41591-021-01407-5.

31. Gandhi M, "Overcaution Carries Its Own Danger to Children," *The Atlantic*, February 27, 2021, https://www.theatlantic.com/ideas/archive/2021/02/vaccines-are-banishing-any-debate-about-reopening

-schools/618155/; Henderson TO, Gandhi M, Hoeg TB, Johnson D, "CDC Misinterpreted Our Research on Opening Schools. It Should Loosen the Rules Now," *USA Today,* March 9, 2021, https://www .usatoday.com/story/opinion/2021/03/09/cdc-school-opening-COVID -rules-guidance-column/4628552001/; Hoeg TB, Henderson TO, Johnson D, Gandhi M, "Our Next National Priority Should Be to Reopen All America's Schools for Full Time In-Person Learning," *The Hill,* March 20, 2021, https://thehill.com/opinion/healthcare/544142 -our-next-national-priority-should-be-to-reopen-all-americas-schools-for/; Bienen L, Happel E, Gandhi M, "Real-World Data, Not Predictions, Should Drive Decisions on COVID-19 and School Opening," STAT, April 23, 2021, https://www.statnews.com/2021/04/23/use-real-world -data-not-predictions-inform-school-opening-decisions/; Noble J, Gandhi M, "Is It Safe to Fully Reopen California Schools? It's Not Unsafe Not To, Says UCSF's Jeanne Noble and Monica Gandhi," *San Francisco Chronicle,* June 4, 2021, https://www.sfchronicle.com/opinion /openforum/article/Is-it-safe-to-fully-reopen-California-schools-1622 4689.php; Hoeg TB, Gandhi M, Johnson D, "We Must Fully Reopen Schools This Fall. Here's How," *New York Times,* June 8, 2021, https:// www.nytimes.com/2021/06/08/opinion/blueprint-reopening-schools. html; Gandhi M, Noble J, "The Pandemic's Toll on Teen Mental Health," *Wall Street Journal,* June 10, 2021, https://www.wsj.com/articles/the -pandemics-toll-on-teen-mental-health-11623344542; Vergales J, Gandhi M, "School Quarantines Keep Too Many Kids at Home—with Barely Any Effect on COVID," *Washington Post,* October 5, 2021, https://www.washingtonpost.com/outlook/2021/10/05/quarantine -COVID-schools-modified-test/; Gandhi M, Johnson D, "A Roadmap to COVID-19 Endemicity in Schools," Smerconish, February 5, 2022, https://www.smerconish.com/exclusive-content/a-roadmap-to-COVID -19-endemicity-in-schools/.

32. Ager P, Eriksson K, Karger E, Nencka P, Thomasson MA, "School Closures During the 1918 Flu Pandemic," *Review of Economics and Statistics* (online), January 25, 2022, https://doi.org/10.1162/rest_a _01170.

33. Taubenberger JK, Morens DM, "1918 Influenza: The Mother of All Pandemics," *Emerging Infectious Diseases* 12, no. 1 (2006): 15–22, https:// doi.org/10.3201/eid1209.05-0979.

34. Bhopal S, Bagaria J, Bhopal R, "Children's Mortality from COVID-19 Compared with All-Deaths and Other Relevant Causes of Death: Epidemiological Information for Decision-Making by Parents, Teachers,

Clinicians and Policymakers," *Public Health* 185 (2020): 19–20, https://doi.org/10.1016/j.puhe.2020.05.047.

35. UNESCO Institute of Statistics, "Global Monitoring of School Closures Caused by COVID-19," accessed July 17, 2022, https://COVID19.uis.unesco.org/global-monitoring-school-closures-COVID19/country-dashboard/.

36. UNESCO Institute of Statistics, "Global Monitoring of School Closures Caused by COVID-19"; Johns Hopkins Coronavirus Resource Center, "Mortality Analyses," accessed August 3, 2022, https://coronavirus.jhu.edu/data/mortality.

37. Adamy J, Overberg P, "Doctors, Once GOP Stalwarts, Now More Likely to Be Democrats," *Wall Street Journal,* October 6, 2019, https://www.wsj.com/articles/doctors-once-gop-stalwarts-now-more-likely-to-be-democrats-11570383523.

38. "Burbio's K–12 School Opening Tracker," last updated June 25, 2022, https://about.burbio.com/school-opening-tracker; Kamenetz A, "The GOP Wants to Be the Education Party. Democrats Have to Fight Back," *Washington Post,* September 7, 2022, https://www.washingtonpost.com/opinions/2022/09/07/democrats-education-republicans-COVID/; Leary A, Hobbs TD, Duehren A, "Trump Administration Pushes for Schools to Reopen," *Wall Street Journal,* July 7, 2020, https://www.wsj.com/articles/trump-administration-pushes-for-schools-to-reopen-11594137764?mod=article_inline.

39. Sacerdote B, Sehgal R, Cook M, "Why Is All COVID-19 News Bad News?," Working Paper no. 28110, National Bureau of Economic Research, November 2020, https://doi.org/10.3386/w28110.

40. Biggs AT, Littlejohn LF, "Revisiting the Initial COVID-19 Pandemic Projections," *Lancet Microbe* 2, no. 3 (2021): e91–e92, https://doi.org/10.1016/S2666-5247(21)00029-X.

41. Shamus KJ, Hall C, Wisely J, "Michigan's COVID-19 Case Rate Is 3rd Worst in US, Schools Go Virtual, Hospitals Fill Up," *Detroit Free Press,* March 25, 2021, https://www.freep.com/story/news/health/2021/03/25/michigan-COVID-19-case-rate-second-worst-in-nation/6986599002/.

42. Bienen et al., "Real-World Data, Not Predictions, Should Drive Decisions on COVID-19 and School Opening."

43. Muller M, "COVID Is Way More Lethal to Kids Than the Flu," Bloomberg, June 3, 2022, https://www.bloomberg.com/news/newsletters/2022-06-03/coronavirus-daily-COVID-is-more-lethal-to-kids-than-the-flu.

44. CDC, "Guidance for Schools and Child Care Programs," last updated October 5, 2022, https://www.cdc.gov/coronavirus/2019-ncov /community/schools-childcare/k-12-childcare-guidance.html; Lovelace B, "Many Patients Hospitalized for Other Ailments Are Also Testing Positive for COVID," NBC News, January 9, 2022, https://www.nbc news.com/health/health-news/omicron-hospital-many-patients -hospitalized-ailments-also-test-positiv-rcna11247.

45. Kelley, "Fact Check: COVID as a Leading Cause of Death in Children," COVID-19 in Georgia, 2022, https://www.COVID-georgia.com /pediatric-news/fact-check-COVID-is-a-leading-cause-of-death-in -children/; Kelley, "COVID vs. Flu for Kids," COVID-19 in Georgia, 2022, https://www.COVID-georgia.com/pediatric-news/COVID -vs-flu-for-kids/; Beck A, Gandhi M, "Adjudicating Reasons for Hospitalization Reveals That Severe Illness from COVID-19 in Children Is Rare," *Hospital Pediatrics* 11, no. 8 (August 1, 2021): e159–e160, doi: 10.1542/hpeds.2021-006084; Kushner LE, Schroeder AR, et al., "'For COVID' or 'With COVID': Classification of SARS-CoV-2 Hospitalizations in Children," *Hospital Pediatrics* 11, no. 8 (August 1, 2021): e151–e156, https://publications.aap.org/hospitalpediatrics/article /11/8/e151/179740/For-COVID-or-With-COVID-Classification-of -SARS-CoV; Webb NE, Osburn TS, "Characteristics of Hospitalized Children Positive for SARS-CoV-2: Experience of a Large Center," *Hospital Pediatrics* 11, no. 8 (August 1, 2021): e133–e141, https:// publications.aap.org/hospitalpediatrics/article/11/8/e133/179737 /Characteristics-of-Hospitalized-Children-Positive.

46. Biggs and Littlejohn, "Revisiting the Initial COVID-19 Pandemic Projections"; Leonhardt D, "COVID Coverage by the U.S. National Media Is an Outlier, a Study Finds," *New York Times,* March 24, 2021, https://www.nytimes.com/2021/03/24/world/COVID-coverage-by-the -us-national-media-is-an-outlier-a-study-finds.html.

47. Portland Public Schools, "January 12 Board Meeting COVID Panel," January 12, 2021, https://drive.google.com/file/d/1mo_Fvrvh0rhOpBU _IZzTLtbCXJv-7cjR/view.

48. "PPS Board of Education Regular Meeting—1/12/21," YouTube, posted by PPS Communications, January 13, 2021, https://www.youtube.com /watch?v=bu-_WS-hOHQ.

49. Oregon Health Authority, "Oregon COVID-19 Case Demographics and Disease Severity Statewide—Summary Table," May 26, 2020, https:// public.tableau.com/app/profile/oregon.health.authority.COVID.19

/viz/OregonCOVID-19CaseDemographicsandDiseaseSeverityState
wide-SummaryTable/DemographicDataSummaryTable.

50. Carbajal E, "States Ranked by COVID-19 Cases: May 5," *Becker's
Hospital Review,* June 1, 2021, https://www.beckershospitalreview.com
/public-health/states-ranked-by-confirmed-COVID-19-cases-july-1.html.

51. Oregon Department of Education, "2020–21 School Status," updated
June 19, 2021, https://www.oregon.gov/ode/students-and-family
/healthsafety/Pages/2020-21-School-Status.aspx.

52. Nuzzo J, "We Don't Need to Close Schools to Fight the Coronavirus,"
New York Times, March 10, 2020, https://www.nytimes.com/2020/03
/10/opinion/coronavirus-school-closing.html.

53. Jenkins R, "LAUSD Just Closed Schools. Ebola Taught Us Why That
May Be Extreme," March 13, 2020, https://www.unicef.org/moldova
/en/stories/op-ed-lausd-just-closed-schools-ebola-taught-us-why-may-be
-extreme; Van Lancker W, Parolin Z, "COVID-19, School Closures, and
Child Poverty: A Social Crisis in the Making," *Lancet Public Health* 5, no.
5 (2020): e243–e244, https://doi.org/10.1016/S2468-2667(20)30084-0;
Lee J, "Mental Health Effects of School Closures During COVID-19,"
Lancet Child and Adolescent Health 4, no. 6 (2020): 421, https://doi
.org/10.1016/S2352-4642(20)30109-7; Fantini MP, Reno C, Biserni GB,
Savoia E, Lanari M, "COVID-19 and the Re-Opening of Schools: A
Policy Maker's Dilemma," *Italian Journal of Pediatrics* 46, no. 1 (2020):
79, https://doi.org/10.1186/s13052-020-00844-1.

54. Rundle AG, Park Y, Herbstman JB, Kinsey EW, Wang YC, "COVID-19–
Related School Closings and Risk of Weight Gain Among Children,"
Obesity 28, no. 6 (2020): 1008–1009, https://doi.org/10.1002
/oby.22813; "Increase Seen in Pediatric BMI During Pandemic, Study
Finds," American Academy of Pediatrics, October 7, 2022, https://
www.aap.org/en/news-room/news-releases/conference-news-releases
/increase-seen-in-pediatric-bmi-during-pandemic-study-finds/.

55. Lee J, "Mental Health Effects of School Closures During COVID-19,"
Lancet Child and Adolescent Health 4, no. 6 (2020): 421, https://doi.org
/10.1016/S2352-4642(20)30109-7.

56. Jenkins, "LAUSD Just Closed Schools. Ebola Taught Us Why That
May Be Extreme."

57. "Suicides on the Rise Amid Stay-at-Home Order, Bay Area Medical
Professionals Say," ABC7 Bay Area, May 21, 2020, https://abc7news.com
/suicide-COVID-19-coronavirus-rates-during-pandemic-death-by
/6201962/.

58. Leeb RT, Bitsko RH, Radhakrishnan L, Martinez P, Njai R, Holland KM, "Mental Health–Related Emergency Department Visits Among Children Aged <18 Years During the COVID-19 Pandemic—United States, January 1–October 17, 2020," *Morbidity and Mortality Weekly Report* 69, no. 45 (2020): 1675–1680, https://doi.org/10.15585/mmwr.mm6945a3.

59. Yard E, Radhakrishnan L, Ballesteros MF, Sheppard M, Gates A, Stein Z, Hartnett K, et al., "Emergency Department Visits for Suspected Suicide Attempts Among Persons Aged 12–25 Years Before and During the COVID-19 Pandemic—United States, January 2019–May 2021," *Morbidity and Mortality Weekly Report* 70, no. 24 (2021): 888–894, https://doi.org/10.15585/mmwr.mm7024e1.

60. Rivera E, "'Their Tank Is Empty': Children's Hospital Colorado Declares a State of Emergency over Kids' Mental Health," KRCC, May 25, 2021, https://www.cpr.org/2021/05/25/COVID-mental-health-childrens-hospital-colorado/; Watson A, "Best of 2021: Children with Psychiatric Needs Are Overwhelming Hospital Emergency Departments in CT," CT Mirror, December 27, 2021, https://ctmirror.org/2021/12/27/best-of-2021-children-with-psychiatric-needs-are-overwhelming-hospital-emergency-departments-in-ct/; Bebinger M, "Kids in Mental Health Crisis Can Languish for Days Inside ERs," NPR, June 23, 2021, https://www.npr.org/sections/health-shots/2021/06/23/1005530668/kids-mental-health-crisis-suicide-teens-er-treatment-boarding.

61. Yard et al., "Emergency Department Visits for Suspected Suicide Attempts Among Persons Aged 12–25 Years Before and During the COVID-19 Pandemic—United States, January 2019–May 2021."

62. Miranda-Mendizabal A, Castellví P, Parés-Badell O, Alayo I, Almenara J, Alonso I, Jesús Blasco M, et al., "Gender Differences in Suicidal Behavior in Adolescents and Young Adults: Systematic Review and Meta-Analysis of Longitudinal Studies," *International Journal of Public Health* 64, no. 2 (2019): 265–283, https://doi.org/10.1007/s00038-018-1196-1.

63. UCSF BCHO, "Mental Health Data," presentation, 2021, https://hividgm.ucsf.edu/sites/hiv.ucsf.edu/files/2021-04/BCHO%20%26%20UCSF%20MB%20-%20Mental%20health%20data.pdf.

64. "U.S. Surgeon General Issues Advisory on Youth Mental Health Crisis Further Exposed by COVID-19 Pandemic," US Department of Health and Human Services, December 7, 2021, https://www.hhs.gov/about/news/2021/12/07/us-surgeon-general-issues-advisory-on-youth-mental-health-crisis-further-exposed-by-COVID-19-pandemic.html.

65. Kuehn B, "CDC Report: Urgent Need to Address Teens' Adverse Experiences During Pandemic," *Journal of the American Medical Association* 328, no. 20 (November 22/29, 2022): 2005, https://jamanetwork.com/journals/jama/fullarticle/2798730.

66. Wang J, Li Y, Musch DC, Wei N, Qi X, Ding G, Li X, et al., "Progression of Myopia in School-Aged Children After COVID-19 Home Confinement," *JAMA Ophthalmology* 139, no. 3 (2021): 293–300, https://doi.org/10.1001/jamaophthalmol.2020.6239; Digitale E, "Youth at Both Ends of Weight Spectrum Challenged by Global Pandemic," Stanford Medicine, March 17, 2021, https://med.stanford.edu/news/all-news/2021/03/pandemic-worsens-weight-woes-among-young-people.html; Woolford SJ, Sidell M, Li X, Else V, Young DR, Resnicow K, Koebnick C, "Changes in Body Mass Index Among Children and Adolescents During the COVID-19 Pandemic," *Journal of the American Medical Association* 326, no. 14 (2021): 1434–1436, https://doi.org/10.1001/jama.2021.15036.

67. WHO, "Immunization Coverage," July 14, 2022, https://www.who.int/news-room/fact-sheets/detail/immunization-coverage; Kaledzi I, "WHO Triggers Measles Outbreak Response," DW, September 12, 2022, https://www.dw.com/en/zimbabwes-measles-outbreak-who-triggers-crisis-response/a-63066598; "Mumbai Measles: India Outbreak Claims 12 Children," BBC News, November 24, 2022, https://www.bbc.com/news/world-asia-india-63739835.

68. United Nations, "Nearly 40 million Children Susceptible to Measles Due to COVID-19 Disruptions," United Nations News, November 23, 2022, https://news.un.org/en/story/2022/11/1131002.

69. Baron EJ, Goldstein EG, Wallace CT, "Suffering in Silence: How COVID-19 School Closures Inhibit the Reporting of Child Maltreatment," *Journal of Public Economics* 190 (2020): 104258, https://doi.org/10.1016/j.jpubeco.2020.104258.

70. Bicker L, "Philippines Sees a Pandemic Boom in Child Sex Abuse," BBC News, November 28, 2022, https://www.bbc.com/news/world-asia-63658818.

71. Korman HTN, O'Keefe B, Repka M, "Missing in the Margins 2021: Revisiting the COVID-19 Attendance Crisis," Bellwether Education Partners, October 21, 2020, https://bellwethereducation.org/publication/missing-margins-estimating-scale-COVID-19-attendance-crisis.

72. Martinez D, Gutierrez G, Romo C, Suarez N, "From the Fields to the Classroom: Inside the Lives of U.S. Agriculture's Youngest Workers," NBC News, September 22, 2020, https://www.nbcnews.com/news

/education/fields-classroom-inside-lives-u-s-agriculture-s-youngest
-workers-n1240159; Klein R, "They Work Full Time. They Attend
School. They're Only Teenagers," *Huffington Post,* September 21, 2020,
https://www.huffpost.com/entry/teenage-breadwinners-pandemic-work
-high-school_n_5f64e367c5b6480e896e3a0c; Kirsch Z, "When Siblings
Become Teachers: It's Not Just Parents Who Find Themselves Thrust into
the Demanding Role of At-Home Educators," The74, April 10, 2020,
https://www.the74million.org/article/when-siblings-become-teachers-its
-not-just-parents-who-find-themselves-thrust-into-the-demanding-role-of
-at-home-educators/; Goodnough A, "As Schools Go Remote, Finding
'Lost' Students Gets Harder," *New York Times,* September 22, 2020,
https://www.nytimes.com/2020/09/22/us/schools-COVID-attendance
.html.

73. Johnson S, "California Teachers Grapple with Grading Nearly a Year
After Initial School Closures," EdSource, February 9, 2021, https://
edsource.org/2021/california-teachers-grapple-with-grading-nearly
-a-year-after-initial-school-closures/648376; "Burbio's K–12 School
Opening Tracker."

74. Johnson, "California Teachers Grapple with Grading Nearly a Year After
Initial School Closures."

75. Woolfolk J, "California Student Test Scores Dismal During COVID
Closures," *Mercury News,* last updated January 13, 2022, https://www
.mercurynews.com/2022/01/07/california-student-test-scores-dismal
-during-COVID-closures/.

76. Rajabi M, "Report 01: COVID-19 Worries, Parents/Carer Stress and
Support Needs, by Child Special Educational Needs and Parent/Carer
Work Status," Co-Space Iran Study, July 10, 2020, http://cospaceoxford
.org/wp-content/uploads/2020/09/Co-SPACE-Iran-Report-1.pdf.

77. Hill F, "The Pandemic Is a Crisis for Students with Special Needs," *The
Atlantic,* April 18, 2020, https://www.theatlantic.com/education/archive
/2020/04/special-education-goes-remote-COVID-19-pandemic/610231/.

78. Dorn E, Hancock B, Sarakatsannis J, "COVID-19 and Student Learning
in the United States: The Hurt Could Last a Lifetime," McKinsey &
Company, June 1, 2020, https://www.mckinsey.com/industries
/education/our-insights/COVID-19-and-student-learning-in-the-united
-states-the-hurt-could-last-a-lifetime.

79. Dorn et al., "COVID-19 and Student Learning in the United States."

80. Adler NE, Newman K, "Socioeconomic Disparities In Health: Pathways
and Policies," *Health Affairs* 21, no. 2 (2002): 60–76, https://doi.org
/10.1377/hlthaff.21.2.60.

81. Goldhaber D, Kane TJ, McEachin A, Morton E, Patterson T, Staiger DO, "The Consequences of Remote and Hybrid Instruction During the Pandemic," Center for Education Policy Research, Harvard University, May 2022, https://cepr.harvard.edu/files/cepr/files/5-4.pdf?m=165169 0491.

82. NAEP, "NAEP Long-Term Trend Assessment Results: Reading and Mathematics," 2022, https://www.nationsreportcard.gov/highlights /ltt/2022/.

83. Filipovic J, "America Has a Problem. We, My Fellow Progressives, Must Admit It," CNN, September 6, 2022, https://www.cnn.com/2022/09 /06/opinions/COVID-school-closures-problem-filipovic/index .html; Kamenetz, "The GOP Wants to Be the Education Party. Democrats Have to Fight Back"; Mervosh S, "The Pandemic Erased Two Decades of Progress in Math and Reading," *New York Times*, September 1, 2022, https://www.nytimes.com/2022/09/01/us/national -test-scores-math-reading-pandemic.html; Chotiner I, "Measuring the Pandemic's Devastating Effect on Schoolchildren," *The New Yorker*, September 8, 2022, https://www.newyorker.com/news/q-and-a /measuring-the-pandemics-devastating-effect-on-schoolchildren.

84. UNICEF, "Pushing More Households and Children into Poverty," 2021, https://data.unicef.org/COVID-19-and-children/.

85. Dworkin SL, Gandhi M, Passano P, eds., *Women's Empowerment and Global Health: A Twenty-First-Century Agenda* (Berkeley: University of California Press, 2017), http://www.jstor.org/stable/10.1525/j .ctv1wxrqm; UNESCO, "Girls' Education and COVID-19: New Factsheet Shows Increased Inequalities for the Education of Adolescent Girls," September 3, 2021, https://gdc.unicef.org/resource/girls -education-and-COVID-19-new-factsheet-shows-increased-inequalities -education.

86. "Even as Omicron Variant Takes Hold, School Closures Must Be a Measure of Last Resort: Statement by UNICEF Executive Director Henrietta Fore," UNICEF, December 17, 2021, https://www.unicef.org /eap/press-releases/even-omicron-variant-takes-hold-school-closures -must-be-measure-last-resort.

87. Goldstein D, "At Head Start, Masks Remain On, Despite C.D.C. Guidelines," *New York Times*, September 7, 2022, https://www.nytimes .com/2022/09/07/us/head-start-masks-toddlers.html; Ladhani SN, "Face Masking for Children—Time to Reconsider," *Journal of Infection* (online), September 25, 2022, doi: 10.1016/j.jinf.2022.09.020; Smelkinson M, Bienen L, Noble J, "The Case Against Masks at School," *The Atlantic*,

January 26, 2022, https://www.theatlantic.com/ideas
/archive/2022/01/kids-masks-schools-weak-science/621133/; Munro
APS, Hughes RC, "Face Coverings Have Little Utility for Young School-
Aged Children," *Archives of Disease in Childhood,* November 3, 2022,
https://adc.bmj.com/content/early/2022/11/03/archdischild-2022
-324809.

88. Esquivel P, "Nearly Half of LAUSD Students Have Been Chronically
Absent This Year, Data Show," *Los Angeles Times,* March 31, 2022,
https://www.latimes.com/california/story/2022-03-31/lausd-students
-chronic-absent-amid-COVID-pandemic.

89. Christakis DA, Van Cleve W, Zimmerman FJ, "Estimation of US
Children's Educational Attainment and Years of Life Lost Associated
with Primary School Closures During the Coronavirus Disease 2019
Pandemic," *JAMA Network Open* 3, no. 11 (2020): e2028786, https://doi.
org/10.1001/jamanetworkopen.2020.28786.

90. Stebbings S, Rotevatn TA, Larsen VB, Surén P, Elstrøm P, Greve-
Isdahl M, Johansen TB, Astrup E, "Experience with Open Schools and
Preschools in Periods of High Community Transmission of COVID-19
in Norway During the Academic Year of 2020/2021," *BMC Public Health*
22, no. 1 (2022): art. 1454, https://doi.org/10.1186/s12889-022
-13868-5.

91. Rotevatn TA, Larsen VB, Johansen TB, Astrup E, Surén P, Greve-Isdahl
M, Telle KE, "Transmission of SARS-CoV-2 in Norwegian Schools
During Academic Year 2020–21: Population Wide, Register Based
Cohort Study," *BMJ Medicine* 1, no. 1 (2021): e000026, https://doi.org
/10.1136/bmjmed-2021-000026.

92. Ulyte A, Radtke T, Abela IA, Haile SR, Ammann P, Berger C,
Trikola A, Fehr J, Puhan MA, Kriemler S, "Evolution of SARS-CoV-2
Seroprevalence and Clusters in School Children from June 2020 to April
2021: Prospective Cohort Study Ciao Corona," *Swiss Medical Weekly* 151
(2021), https://doi.org/10.4414/SMW.2021.w30092.

93. Viner RM, Mytton OT, Bonell C, "Susceptibility to SARS-CoV-2
Infection Among Children and Adolescents Compared with Adults:
A Systematic Review and Meta-Analysis," *JAMA Pediatrics* 175, no. 2
(2020): 143–156, https://doi.org/10.1001/jamapediatrics.2020.4573;
Larosa E, Djuric O, Cassinadri M, Cilloni S, Bisaccia E, Vicentini M,
Venturelli F, et al., "Secondary Transmission of COVID-19 in Preschool
and School Settings in Northern Italy After Their Reopening in
September 2020: A Population-Based Study," *Eurosurveillance* 25, no. 49

(2020): 2001911, https://doi.org/10.2807/1560-7917.ES.2020.25.49
.2001911.

94. Vlachos J, Hertegård E, Svaleryd HB, "The Effects of School Closures on
SARS-CoV-2 Among Parents and Teachers," *Proceedings of the National
Academy of Sciences* 118, no. 9 (2021): e2020834118, https://doi.org/10
.1073/pnas.2020834118.

95. Lewis SJ, Munro APS, Smith GD, Pollock AM, "Closing Schools Is
Not Evidence Based and Harms Children," *BMJ* 372, no. 521 (2021):
e2020834118, https://doi.org/10.1136/bmj.n521; Forbes H, Morton
CE, Bacon S, McDonald HI, Minassian C, Brown JP, Rentsch CT, et
al., "Association Between Living with Children and Outcomes from
COVID-19: OpenSAFELY Cohort Study of 12 Million Adults in
England," *BMJ* 372, no. 628 (2021), https://doi.org/10.1136/bmj.n628.

96. Kim J, Choe YJ, Lee J, Park YJ, Park O, Han MS, Kim JH, Choi EH,
"Role of Children in Household Transmission of COVID-19," *Archives of
Disease in Childhood* 106 (2020): 709–711, https://doi.org/10.1136
/archdischild-2020-319910.

97. Ertem Z, Schechter-Perkins E, Oster E, van der Berg P, Epshtein I,
Chaiyakunapruk N, Wilson F, et al., "The Impact of School Opening
Model on SARS-CoV-2 Community Incidence and Mortality," *Nature
Medicine* 27 (2021): 2120–2126, https://doi.org/10.1038/s41591-021
-01563-8.

98. Zimmerman KO, Akinboyo IC, et al., "Incidence and Secondary
Transmission of SARS-CoV-2 Infections in Schools," *Pediatrics* 147, no. 4
(April 1, 2021): e2020048090, https://publications.aap.org/pediatrics
/article/147/4/e2020048090/180871/Incidence-and-Secondary
-Transmission-of-SARS-CoV-2.

99. Engzell P, Frey A, Verhagen MD, "Learning Loss Due to School Closures
During the COVID-19 Pandemic," *Proceedings of the National Academy of
Sciences* 118, no. 17 (2021): e2022376118, https://doi.org/10.1073/pnas
.2022376118.

100. Vira EG, Skoog T, "Swedish Middle School Students' Psychosocial Well-
Being During the COVID-19 Pandemic: A Longitudinal Study," *SSM—
Population Health* 16 (2021): 100942, https://doi.org/10.1016/j.ssmph
.2021.100942.

101. Sachs JD, Karim SSA, Aknin L, Allen J, Brosbøl K, Colombo F, Cuevas
Barron G, et al., "The Lancet Commission on Lessons for the Future
from the COVID-19 Pandemic," *Lancet* 400, no. 10359 (2022): 1224–
1280, https://doi.org/10.1016/S0140-6736(22)01585-9.

102. Sachs et al., "The Lancet Commission on Lessons for the Future from the COVID-19 Pandemic."

103. Azevedo JP, Rogers H, Ahlgren E, Cloutier MH, Chakroun B, Chang GC, Mizunoya S, Reuge N, Brossard M, Bergmann JL, "The State of the Global Education Crisis: A Path to Recovery," World Bank Group, December 10, 2021, http://documents.worldbank.org/curated/en/41699 1638768297704/The-State-of-the-Global-Education-Crisis-A-Path-to -Recovery.

104. UN, "Education Summit Offers 'Once-in-a-Lifetime' Chance to Recover Learning Losses, Advance Badly Off-Track Goals and Rethink Education Systems," press release, September 16, 2022, https://www.un.org /sustainabledevelopment/blog/2022/09/press-release-education-summit -offers-once-in-a-lifetime-chance-to-recover-learning-losses-advance -badly-off-track-goals-and-rethink-education-systems/.

105. "UN Chief Warns Education Becoming 'Great Divider,'" France 24, September 19, 2022, https://www.france24.com/en/live-news/2022 0919-un-chief-warns-education-becoming-great-divider.

106. Eldred SM, "It's a Bleak 'Day of the Girl' Because of the Pandemic. But No One's Giving Up Hope," NPR, October 11, 2022, https://www.npr .org/sections/goatsandsoda/2022/10/11/1127313745/its-a-bleak-day-of -the-girl-because-of-the-pandemic-but-no-ones-giving-up-hope.

107. UNICEF, "COVID-19: Scale of Education Loss 'Nearly Insurmountable,' Warns UNICEF," January 23, 2022, https://www .unicef.org/press-releases/COVID19-scale-education-loss-nearly -insurmountable-warns-unicef.

108. UNICEF, "COVID-19: Scale of Education Loss 'Nearly Insurmountable,' Warns UNICEF."

109. Sachs et al., "The Lancet Commission on Lessons for the Future from the COVID-19 Pandemic."

110. "COVID Learning Loss Has Been a Global Disaster," *The Economist,* July 7, 2022, https://www.economist.com/international/2022/07/07/COVID -learning-loss-has-been-a-global-disaster.

111. LaMesa A, "How European Schools Stay Open," *The Grade,* December 8, 2020, https://kappanonline.org/how-european-schools-stay-open-lamesa -russo/.

112. European Centre for Disease Prevention and Control, "COVID-19 in Children and the Role of School Settings in Transmission—Second Update," July 8, 2021, https://www.ecdc.europa.eu/sites/default/files /documents/COVID-19-in-children-and-the-role-of-school-settings -in-transmission-second-update.pdf.

113. Khullar D, "Living with Our Pandemic Trade-Offs," *The New Yorker,* September 18, 2022, https://www.newyorker.com/magazine/2022/09/26 /living-with-our-pandemic-trade-offs.

114. Office of the Prime Minister, "The Norwegian Government's Management of the Coronavirus Pandemic—Part 2—Summary in English," 2022, https://www.regjeringen.no/contentassets/d0b6 1f6e1d1b40d1bb92ff9d9b60793d/en-gb/pdfs/nou202220220005000 engpdfs.pdf; Dutch Safety Board, "Corona Response. Part 2: September 2020–July 2021," October 12, 2022, https://www.onderzoeksraad.nl /en/aanpak-coronacrisis-deel2; UK Parliament, "The Government's Response to Coronavirus," 2020, https://committees.parliament.uk /work/192/the-governments-response-to-coronavirus/publications/; "Managing the COVID-19-Crisis: Report Delivered to the Standing Orders Committee of the Danish Parliament January 2021," Folketinget, January 2021, https://www.thedanishparliament.dk/- /media/sites/ft/pdf/publikationer/engelske-publikationer-pdf /managing-the-COVID19-crisis.ashx; Shergold P, Broadbent J, Marshall I, Varghese P, "Fault Lines: An Independent Review into Australia's Response to COVID-19," Paul Ramsay Foundation, October 20, 2022, https://www.smh.com.au/interactive/hub/media/tearout-excerpt /10774/Independent-Review-into-Australia's-response-to-COVID -19.pdf.

115. Daignault M, Gandhi M, "Omicron, Delta, and the Need for More Accurate Hospitalization Data," Smerconish, January 6, 2022, https:// www.smerconish.com/exclusive-content/omicron-delta-and-the-need-for -more-accurate-hospitalization-data/.

116. McCluskey PD, "Why This Wave of COVID Hospitalizations in Mass. Is Different," WBUR, June 1, 2022, https://www.wbur.org/news/2022 /06/01/COVID-hospitals-massachusetts-different-wave.

117. Moffa MA, Shively NR, Carr DR, Bremmer DN, Buchanan C, Trienski TL, Jacobs MW, Saini V, Walsh TL, "Description of Hospitalizations Due to the Severe Acute Respiratory Syndrome Coronavirus 2 Omicron Variant Based on Vaccination Status," *Open Forum Infectious Diseases* 9, no. 9 (2022), https://doi.org/10.1093/ofid/ofac438.

118. Department of Health and Social Care, "Regular Asymptomatic Testing Paused in Additional Settings," August 24, 2022, https://www.gov.uk /government/news/regular-asymptomatic-testing-paused-in-additional -settings.

119. Young BC, Eyre DW, Kendrick S, White W, Smith S, Beveridge G, Nonnenmacher T, et al., "Daily Testing for Contacts of Individuals with

SARS-CoV-2 Infection and Attendance and SARS-CoV-2 Transmission in English Secondary Schools and Colleges: An Open-Label, Cluster-Randomised Trial," *Lancet* 398, no. 10307 (2021): 1217–1229, https://doi.org/10.1016/S0140-6736(21)01908-5; Abaluck J, Kwong LH, Styczynski A, Haque A, Kabir A, Bates-Jefferys E, Crawford E, et al., "Impact of Community Masking on COVID-19: A Cluster-Randomized Trial in Bangladesh," *Science* 375, no. 6577 (2021): eabi9069, https://doi.org/10.1126/science.abi9069.

120. García E, Weiss E, "Low Relative Pay and High Incidence of Moonlighting Play a Role in the Teacher Shortage, Particularly in High-Poverty Schools," Economic Policy Institute, May 9, 2019, https://epi.org/161908; Subaru of America, "Teachers Spending More Out of Pocket on School Supplies Than Ever Before," NewsDirect, August 18, 2021, https://newsdirect.com/news/teachers-spending-more-out-of-pocket-on-school-supplies-than-ever-before-852951135; Natanson H, "'Never Seen It This Bad': America Faces Catastrophic Teacher Shortage," *Washington Post*, August 3, 2022, https://www.washingtonpost.com/education/2022/08/03/school-teacher-shortage/; Gonzalez L, Brown M, Slate J, "Teachers Who Left the Teaching Profession: A Qualitative Understanding," *Qualitative Report* 13, no. 1 (2008): 1–11, https://doi.org/10.46743/2160-3715/2008.1601.

121. Natanson, "'Never Seen It This Bad': America Faces Catastrophic Teacher Shortage"; Nimmo T, "Combating Teacher Burnout: Nationwide Teacher Shortage Has Experts Worried About Future of Education," WPCO, August 2, 2022, https://www.wcpo.com/news/local-news/campbell-county/newport-community/combating-teacher-burnout-nationwide-teacher-shortage-has-experts-worried-about-future-of-education; Gertler J, "Teacher Shortage Straining School Districts Like MSCS," WREG, August 1, 2022, https://wreg.com/news/local/teacher-shortage-straining-school-districts-like-mscs/; Bergan S, Campbell M, Hennessy J, "Teacher Shortages Spurring 4-Day Weeks, Hefty Sign-On Bonuses," KCTV, August 4, 2022, https://www.kctv5.com/2022/08/04/teacher-shortages-spurring-4-day-weeks-hefty-sign-on-bonuses/.

122. Bienen L, "It's Time to Do Something About America's Failure to Recognize Children's Rights," *Sensible Medicine,* August 14, 2022, https://sensiblemed.substack.com/p/its-time-to-do-something-about-americas.

123. Swedish Constitution, 1974 (rev. 2012), Article 2, https://www.constituteproject.org/constitution/Sweden_2012; Adolphsen C, "Constitutional Rights for Danish Children," in *Children's Constitutional*

Rights in the Nordic Countries, ed. Haugli T, Nylund A, Sigurdsen R, Bendiksen LRL, 120–130 (Nijhoff: Brill, 2019), https://doi.org/10.1163/9789004382817_008.

124. "Norway Constitutional and Legal Foundations," StateUniversity.com Education Encyclopedia, accessed August 4, 2022, https://education.stateuniversity.com/pages/1122/Norway-CONSTITUTIONAL-LEGAL-FOUNDATIONS.html.

125. "Article 14—Right to Education," *Official Journal of the European Union,* December 14, 2007, https://fra.europa.eu/en/eu-charter/article/14-right-education.

126. Queensland Human Rights Commission, "Section 36 of the Human Rights Act 2019," https://www.qhrc.qld.gov.au/__data/assets/pdf_file/0006/19905/QHRC_factsheet_HRA_s36.pdf.

127. Gandhi and Johnson, "A Roadmap to COVID-19 Endemicity in Schools."

128. Allen JG, Ibrahim AM, "Indoor Air Changes and Potential Implications for SARS-CoV-2 Transmission," *Journal of the American Medical Association* 325, no. 20 (2021): 2112–2113, https://doi.org/10.1001/jama.2021.5053; Corsi R, Miller SL, VanRy MG, Marr LC, Cadet LR, Pollock NR, Michaels D, et al., "Designing Infectious Disease Resilience into School Buildings Through Improvements to Ventilation and Air Cleaning," *Lancet* COVID-19 Commission Task Force on Safe Work, Safe School, and Safe Travel, April 2021, https://static1.squarspace.com/static/5ef3652ab722df11fcb2ba5d/t/60a3d1251fcec67243e91119/1621348646314/Safe+Work+TF+Desigining+infectious+disease+resilience+April+2021.pdf.

129. Children's Hospital of Philadelphia, "Guidance for Updated COVID-19 School Mitigation Plans for Academic Year 2022–23," August 2022, https://policylab.chop.edu/sites/default/files/pdf/publications/PolicyLab-CHOP-Guidance-for-Updated-COVID-19-School-Mitigation-Plans-2022-23.pdf.

130. "'In-School Transmission Extremely Rare' as Mass. Starts New COVID-19 at Home Tests for Students, Teachers," WCVB, January 18, 2022, https://www.msn.com/en-us/news/us/in-school-transmission-extremely-rare-as-mass-starts-new-COVID-19-at-home-tests-for-students-teachers/ar-AASTmTP?ocid=winp-st.

131. Action for Healthy Kids, "Time to Eat," accessed August 4, 2022, https://www.actionforhealthykids.org/activity/time-to-eat/.

132. Gandhi M, Marr LC, "Uniting Infectious Disease and Physical Science Principles on the Importance of Face Masks for COVID-19," *Med* 2

(2021): 21–32, https://doi.org/10.1016/j.medj.2020.12.008; Khazan O, "One-Way Masking Works," *The Atlantic,* January 10, 2022, https:// www.theatlantic.com/politics/archive/2022/01/does-it-help-wear-mask -if-no-one-else/621177/.

133. NAEP, "Largest Score Declines in NAEP Mathematics at Grades 4 and 8 Since Initial Assessments in 1990," October 2022, https://www.nations reportcard.gov/highlights/mathematics/2022/.

CHAPTER 6: THE NEED FOR GLOBAL EQUITY
IN COVID-19 VACCINES AND TREATMENTS

1. Mathieu E, Ritchie H, Rodés-Guirao L, Appel C, Giattino C, Hasell H, Macdonald B, Dattani S, Beltekian D, Ortiz-Ospina E, Roser R, "Coronavirus Pandemic (COVID-19)," Our World in Data, 2020, https://ourworldindata.org/COVID-vaccinations.

2. Hammerman A, Sergienko R, Friger M, Beckenstein T, Peretz A, Netzer D, Yaron S, Arbel R, "Effectiveness of the BNT162b2 Vaccine After Recovery from COVID-19," *New England Journal of Medicine* 386 (2022): 1221–1229, https://www.nejm.org/doi/full/10.1056/nejmoa 2119497; Gandhi M, "Immunity Against the Omicron Variant from Vaccination, Recovery, or Both," *Clinical Infectious Diseases* 75, no. 1 (2022): 672–674, https://doi.org/10.1093/cid/ciac172.

3. Gandhi M, "The Most Important Thing Rich Countries Can Do to Help India Fight COVID-19," *Time,* May 4, 2021, https://time.com/6046096 /india-COVID-19-vaccine-patents/; Diamond D, Stein J, "White House Is Split over How to Vaccinate the World," *Washington Post,* April 30, 2021, https://www.washingtonpost.com/health/2021/04/30/biden -administration-debates-waiving-vaccine-patents/; "Tracking Coronavirus in India: Latest Map and Case Count," *New York Times,* updated October 18, 2022, https://www.nytimes.com/interactive/2021 /world/india-COVID-cases.html; WTO, "TRIPS—Trade-Related Aspects of Intellectual Property Rights," 2022, https://www.wto.org /english/tratop_e/trips_e/trips_e.htm; Thompson M, et al., "Interim Estimates of Vaccine Effectiveness of BNT162b2 and mRNA-1273 COVID-19 Vaccines in Preventing SARS-CoV-2 Infection Among Health Care Personnel, First Responders, and Other Essential and Frontline Workers—Eight U.S. Locations, December 2020–March

2021," *Morbidity and Mortality Weekly Report* 70 (2021): 495–500, http://dx.doi.org/10.15585/mmwr.mm7013e3.

4. Ward C, Yeung J, "As India's Crematoriums Overflow with COVID Victims, Pyres Burn Through the Night," CNN, May 1, 2021, https://www.cnn.com/2021/04/29/india/india-COVID-deaths-crematoriums-intl-hnk-dst/index.html; Maxouris C, "More Relaxed CDC Coronavirus Guidelines Could Come Soon, Fauci Says," CNN, April 29, 2021, https://www.cnn.com/2021/04/28/health/us-coronavirus-wednesday/index.html.

5. Brennan Z, "BioNTech Makes a Splash with $10B+ Projection for 2021 COVID-19 Vaccine Sales," EndpointsNews, March 30, 2021, https://endpts.com/biontech-makes-a-splash-with-10b-projection-for-2021-COVID-19-vaccine-sales/.

6. WTO, "Waiver from Certain Provisions of the TRIPS Agreement for the Prevention, Containment and Treatment of COVID-19," December 2, 2020, https://docs.wto.org/dol2fe/Pages/SS/directdoc.aspx?filename=q:/IP/C/W669.pdf.

7. "Coronavirus News March 5: Highlights," *India Today,* March 5, 2021, https://www.indiatoday.in/coronavirus-COVID-19-outbreak/story/coronavirus-live-updates-march-5-COVID-vaccine-india-world-daily-cases-deaths-1775790-2021-03-05; Ubl S, et al., "Letter to President Joseph Biden from Pharmaceutical Companies," PhRMA, March 5, 2021, https://patentdocs.typepad.com/files/2021-03-05-phrma-letter.pdf.

8. Gandhi M, "Four Ways HIV Activists Saved Lives During COVID," *Newsweek,* April 12, 2021, https://www.newsweek.com/four-ways-hiv-activists-saved-lives-during-COVID-opinion-1582504; Vachani S, "South Africa and the AIDS Epidemic," *Sage Journals* 29, no. 1 (2004): 101–109, https://journals.sagepub.com/doi/pdf/10.1177/0256090920040109.

9. "HIV and AIDS–United States, 1981–2000," *Morbidity and Mortality Weekly Report* 50, no. 21 (2001): 430–434, https://www.cdc.gov/mmwr/preview/mmwrhtml/mm5021a2.htm.

10. "Pfizer Revenue 2010–2022: PFE," Macrotrends, https://www.macrotrends.net/stocks/charts/PFE/pfizer/revenue; James JS, "Fluconazole: Pfizer Asked to Lower Africa Price," *AIDS Treatment News* 17, no. 339 (2000): 5–6, https://pubmed.ncbi.nlm.nih.gov/12870451/.

11. Shroufi A, et al., "Ending Deaths from HIV-Related Cryptococcal Meningitis by 2030," *Lancet Infectious Diseases* 21, no. 1 (2021): P16–P18,

https://www.thelancet.com/journals/laninf/article/PIIS1473-3099
(20)30909-9/fulltext.

12. James, "Fluconazole: Pfizer Asked to Lower Africa Price."

13. Vachani, "South Africa and the AIDS Epidemic."

14. Smith NC, Vachani S, "When the Price Isn't Right," London Business
School, June 1, 2005, https://www.london.edu/think/when-the-price
-isnt-right.

15. UNAIDS, "Report on the Global HIV/AIDS Epidemic," June 2000,
https://data.unaids.org/pub/report/2000/2000_gr_en.pdf.

16. WTO, "Overview: The TRIPS Agreement," https://www.wto.org
/english/tratop_e/trips_e/intel2_e.htm.

17. 't Hoen et al., "Driving a Decade of Change: HIV/AIDS, Patents and
Access to Medicines for All," *Journal of the International AIDS
Society* 14, no. 1 (2011): 15, https://onlinelibrary.wiley.com/doi/full
/10.1186/1758-2652-14-15.

18. 't Hoen E, Berger J, Calmy A, Moon S, "Driving a Decade of Change:
HIV/AIDS, Patents and Access to Medicines for All."

19. UNAIDS, "In Danger: UNAIDS Global AIDS Update 2022," July 27,
2022, https://www.unaids.org/en/resources/documents/2022/in-danger
-global-aids-update.

20. Holder J, "Tracking Coronavirus Vaccinations Around the World," *New
York Times,* accessed October 10, 2022, https://www.nytimes.com
/interactive/2021/world/COVID-vaccinations-tracker.html.

21. UN, "Secretary-General Calls Vaccine Equity Biggest Moral Test for
Global Community, as Security Council Considers Equitable Availability
of Doses," press release, February 17, 2021, https://press.un.org/en/2021
/sc14438.doc.htm.

22. Watson O, et al., "Global Impact of the First Year of COVID-19
Vaccination: A Mathematical Modeling Study," *Lancet Infectious Diseases*
22, no. 9 (2022): P1293–P1302, https://www.thelancet.com/journals
/laninf/article/PIIS1473-3099(22)00320-6/fulltext.

23. "35 Generic Manufacturers Sign Agreements with MPP to Produce
Low-Cost, Generic Versions of Pfizer's Oral COVID-19 Treatment
Nirmatrelvir in Combination with Ritonavir for Supply in 95 Low- and
Middle-Income Countries," Medicines Patent Pool, March 17, 2022,
https://medicinespatentpool.org/news-publications-post/35-generic
-manufacturers-sign-agreements-with-mpp-to-produce-low-cost
-generic-versions-of-pfizers-oral-COVID-19-treatment-nirmatrelvir-in
-combination-with-ritonavir-for-supply-in-95-low-and.

24. Shadlen K, "Accelerating Pooled Licensing of Medicines to Enhance Global Production and Equitable Access," *Lancet* 400, no. 10352 (2022): 632–634, https://www.ncbi.nlm.nih.gov/pmc/articles/PMC9270061/.

25. Steenhuysen J, Roy M, "WHO Lays Out Plan to Emerge from Emergency Phase of Pandemic," Reuters, March 30, 2022, https://www.reuters.com/business/healthcare-pharmaceuticals/who-lays-out-plan-emerge-emergency-phase-pandemic-2022-03-30/.

26. Butt A, et al., "COVID-19 Disease Severity in Persons Infected with Omicron BA.1 and BA.2 Sublineages and Association with Vaccination Status," *JAMA Internal Medicine* 182, no. 10 (2022): 1097–1099, https://jamanetwork.com/journals/jamainternalmedicine/fullarticle/2795326.

27. Ng OT, et al., "Analysis of COVID-19 Incidence and Severity Among Adults Vaccinated with 2-Dose mRNA COVID-19 or Inactivated SARS-CoV-2 Vaccines with and Without Boosters in Singapore," *JAMA Network Open* 5, no. 8 (2022): e2228900, https://jamanetwork.com/journals/jamanetworkopen/fullarticle/2795654.

28. Buckner C, et al., "Recent SARS-CoV-2 Infection Abrogates Antibody and B-Cell Responses to Booster Vaccination," *medRxiv,* August 31, 2022, https://www.medrxiv.org/content/10.1101/2022.08.30.22279344v1.

29. Arbel R, et al., "Nirmatrelvir Use and Severe COVID-19 Outcomes During the Omicron Surge," *New England Journal of Medicine* 387 (2022): 790–798, https://www.nejm.org/doi/full/10.1056/NEJMoa2204919.

30. Palm AK, Henry C, "Remembrance of Things Past: Long-Term B Cell Memory After Infection and Vaccination," *Frontiers in Immunology* 10 (2019): 1787, https://www.frontiersin.org/articles/10.3389/fimmu.2019.01787/full.

31. Barouch D, "COVID-19 Vaccines—Immunity, Variants, Boosters," *New England Journal of Medicine* 387 (2022): 1011–1020, https://www.nejm.org/doi/full/10.1056/NEJMra2206573.

32. Gandhi M, Daignault M, "We Need to Clarify the Goal of Our COVID Booster Strategy," MedPage Today, March 30, 2022, https://www.medpagetoday.com/opinion/second-opinions/97948; Doron S, Gandhi M, "New Boosters Are Here! Who Should Receive Them and When?," *Lancet Infectious Diseases* (online), October 27, 2022, https://doi.org/10.1016/S1473-3099(22)00688-0.

33. Doron and Gandhi, "New Boosters Are Here! Who Should Receive Them and When?"

CHAPTER 7: A POST-PANDEMIC PLAYBOOK

1. Halperin D, et al., "Revisiting COVID-19 Policies: 10 Evidence-Based Recommendations for Where to Go from Here," *BMC Public Health,* November 13, 2021, https://bmcpublichealth.biomedcentral.com /articles/10.1186/s12889-021-12082-z.

2. CDC, "1918 Pandemic (H1N1 Virus)," March 30, 2019, https://www .cdc.gov/flu/pandemic-resources/1918-pandemic-h1n1.html; CDC, "Measles History," November 5, 2020, https://www.cdc.gov/measles /about/history.html.

3. CDC, "Measles History."

4. Downie AW, "Infection and Immunity in Smallpox," *Lancet* 257, no. 6653 (1951): 419–422, https://www.thelancet.com/journals/lancet /article/PIIS0140-6736(51)92026-0/fulltext.

5. Park A, Ducharme J, "Vaccine Scientists: Heroes of the Year 2021," *Time,* December 13, 2021, https://time.com/heroes-of-the-year-2021-vaccine -scientists/; Graham B, Sullivan N, "Emerging Viral Diseases from a Vaccinology Perspective: Preparing for the Next Pandemic," *Nature Immunology,* December 14, 2017, https://www.nature.com/articles/s415 90-017-0007-9.

6. Dolgin E, "The Tangled History of mRNA Vaccines," *Nature,* September 14, 2021, https://www.nature.com/articles/d41586-021-02483-w.

7. Klein N, Lewis N, Goddard K, "Surveillance for Adverse Events After COVID-19 mRNA Vaccination," *Journal of the American Medical Association,* September 3, 2021, https://jamanetwork.com/journals /jama/fullarticle/2784015; Kanwal S, "Number of COVID-19 Vaccine Doses Administered in India as of September 1, 2022, by Type," Statista, September 1, 2022, https://www.statista.com/statistics/1248301 /india-COVID-19-vaccines-administered-by-vaccine-type/.

8. Wang H, et al., "Estimating Excess Mortality Due to the COVID-19 Pandemic: A Systematic Analysis of COVID-19-Related Mortality, 2020–21," *Lancet* 399, no. 10334 (2022): 1513–1536, https://www .thelancet.com/article/S0140-6736(21)02796-3/.

9. Johns Hopkins Coronavirus Resource Center, "Vaccines," 2022, https:// coronavirus.jhu.edu/vaccines#:~:text=As%20Africa%20goes%20 unvaccinated%2C%20U.S.,U.S.%20population%20is%20fully%20 vaccinated; Simmons-Duffin S, Nakajima K, "This Is How Many Lives Could Have Been Saved with COVID Vaccinations in Each State," NPR, May 13, 2022, https://www.npr.org/sections/health-shots/2022/05/13

/1098071284/this-is-how-many-lives-could-have-been-saved-with
-COVID-vaccinations-in-each-sta; Flam F, "The Tragedy of Avoidable
COVID Deaths," Bloomberg, December 3, 2022, https://www
.bloomberg.com/opinion/articles/2022-12-03/low-us-covid-vaccine
-rates-led-to-high-death-rates-during-delta-omicron.

10. Gandhi M, "Want to Motivate Vaccinations? Message Optimism, Not
Doom," Leaps, February 6, 2021, https://leaps.org/want-to-motivate
-vaccinations-focus-on-the-reasons-for-optimism-not-continual-doom/.

11. Gandhi M, Havlir D, "The Time for Universal Masking of the Public
for Coronavirus Disease 2019 Is Now," *Open Forum Infectious Diseases*
7, no. 4 (2020): ofaa131, https://pubmed.ncbi.nlm.nih.gov/32346544/;
Leonhardt D, "Why Masks Work, but Mandates Haven't," *New York
Times,* May 31, 2022, https://www.nytimes.com/2022/05/31/briefing
/masks-mandates-us-COVID.html.

12. Potts M, Halperin DT, Kirby D, Swidler A, Marseille E, Klausner JD, et
al., "Public Health: Reassessing HIV Prevention," *Science* 320, no. 5877
(2008): 749–750, https://doi.org/10.1126/science.1153843; Kutscher E,
Greene RE, "A Harm-Reduction Approach to Coronavirus Disease 2019
(COVID-19)—Safer Socializing," *JAMA Health Forum* 1, no. 6 (2020):
e200656, https://doi.org/10.1001/jamahealthforum.2020.0656; Marcus J,
"Quarantine Fatigue Is Real," *The Atlantic,* May 11, 2020, https://
www.theatlantic.com/ideas/archive/2020/05/quarantine-fatigue-real-and
-shaming-people-wont-help/611482/.

13. Kutscher and Greene, "A Harm-Reduction Approach to Coronavirus
Disease 2019 (COVID-19)—Safer Socializing"; Marcus, "Quarantine
Fatigue Is Real"; Escandón K, Rasmussen AL, Bogoch II, Murray EJ,
Escandón K, Popescu SV, et al., "COVID-19 False Dichotomies and
a Comprehensive Review of the Evidence Regarding Public Health,
COVID-19 Symptomatology, SARS-CoV-2 Transmission, Mask
Wearing, and Reinfection," *BMC Infectious Diseases* 21, no. 1 (2021):
710, https://doi.org/10.1186/s12879-021-06357-4; Barocas J, Gandhi M,
"Harm Reduction Principles Can Help Us Restore Trust in Public Health
Messaging on COVID-19," *BMJ Opinion* (blog), December 15, 2020,
https://blogs.bmj.com/bmj/2020/12/15/harm-reduction-principles-can
-help-us-restore-trust-in-public-health-messaging-on-COVID-19/.

14. Normile D, "Japan Ends Its COVID-19 State of Emergency," *Science,*
May 26, 2020, https://doi.org/10.1126/science.abd0092.

15. Escandón et al., "COVID-19 False Dichotomies and a Comprehensive
Review of the Evidence Regarding Public Health, COVID-19
Symptomatology, SARS-CoV-2 Transmission, Mask Wearing, and

Reinfection"; Halperin DT, "Coping with COVID-19: Learning from Past Pandemics to Avoid Pitfalls and Panic," *Global Health: Science and Practice* 8, no. 2 (2020): 155–165, https://doi.org/10.9745/GHSP-D-20 -00189; Barocas J, Gonsalves G, "Make It Easier to Stay Safe from COVID-19, Instead of Shaming and Punishing People," *USA Today,* December 7, 2020, https://www.usatoday.com/story/opinion/2020/12 /07/stop-COVID-shaming-punishing-give-incentives-to-stay-safe -column/3812823001/; Marcus J, Martin M, "Epidemiologist on Why 'Pandemic Shaming' Isn't Working," NPR, December 19, 2020, https:// www.npr.org/2020/12/19/948403401/epidemiologist-on-why-pandemic -shaming-isn-t-working.

16. Pavli A, Maltezou HC, "COVID-19 Vaccine Passport for Safe Resumption of Travel," *Journal of Travel Medicine* 28, no. 4 (2021): taab079, https://doi.org/10.1093/jtm/taab079; Sharun K, Tiwari R, Dhama K, Rabaan AA, Alhumaid S, "COVID-19 Vaccination Passport: Prospects, Scientific Feasibility, and Ethical Concerns," *Human Vaccines and Immunotherapeutics* 17, no. 11 (2021): 4108–4111, https://doi.org /10.1080/21645515.2021.1953350; Dye C, Mills MC, "COVID-19 Vaccination Passports," *Science* 371, no. 6535 (2021): 1184, https://doi .org/10.1126/science.abi5245.

17. Cevik M, Marcus JL, Buckee C, Smith TC, "SARS-CoV-2 Transmission Dynamics Should Inform Policy," *Clinical Infectious Diseases* 73, supp. 2 (2021): S170–S176, https://doi.org/10.1093/cid/ciaa1442.

18. Miller AM, "Stop Shaming People for Going Outside. The Risks Are Generally Low, and the Benefits Are Endless," *Business Insider,* June 10, 2020, https://www.businessinsider.com/you-can-still-go-outside-while -quarantining-sheltering-in-place-2020-4; Popkin G, "Don't Cancel the Outdoors. We Need It to Stay Sane," *Washington Post,* March 24, 2020, https://www.washingtonpost.com/outlook/2020/03/24/dont-cancel -outdoors-we-need-them-stay-sane/; DeCosta-Klipa N, "UMass Amherst Is Prohibiting Outdoor Exercise During Its Lockdown. But Why?," *Boston Globe,* February 11, 2021, https://www.boston.com/news /coronavirus/2021/02/11/umass-amherst-lockdown-outdoor-exercise; Bote J, "Officers at Dorms, Outdoor Exercise Ban: UC Berkeley Extends Dorm Lockdown with Stricter Mandates," SF Gate, February 9, 2021, https://www.sfgate.com/education/article/Police-dorms-outdoor -exercise-UC-Berkeley-lockdown-15937294.php; Tufekci Z, "Keep the Parks Open," *The Atlantic,* April 7, 2020, https://www.theatlantic.com /health/archive/2020/04/closing-parks-ineffective-pandemic-theater /609580/; Tufekci Z, "Scolding Beachgoers Isn't Helping," *The Atlantic,*

July 4, 2020, https://www.theatlantic.com/health/archive/2020/07/it -okay-go-beach/613849/.

19. Escandón et al., "COVID-19 False Dichotomies and a Comprehensive Review of the Evidence Regarding Public Health, COVID-19 Symptomatology, SARS-CoV-2 Transmission, Mask Wearing, and Reinfection"; Leclerc QJ, Fuller NM, Knight LE, Funk S, Knight GM, "What Settings Have Been Linked to SARS-CoV-2 Transmission Clusters?," *Wellcome Open Research* 5, no. 83 (2020), https://doi.org /10.12688/wellcomeopenres.15889.2; Qian H, Miao T, Liu L, Zheng X, Luo D, Li Y, "Indoor Transmission of SARS-CoV-2," *Indoor Air* 31, no. 3 (2021): 639–645, https://doi.org/10.1111/ina.12766; McGreevy R, "Outdoor Transmission Accounts for 0.1% of State's COVID-19 Cases," *Irish Times,* April 5, 2021, https://www.irishtimes.com/news/ireland /irish-news/outdoor-transmission-accounts-for-0-1-of-state-s-COVID -19-cases-1.4529036; Lakha F, Rudge JW, Holt H, "Rapid Synthesis of Evidence on Settings Which Have Been Associated with SARS-CoV-2 Transmission Clusters," July 1, 2020, https://superspreadingdatabase .github.io/Evidence_on_clusters_final.pdf; Fouda B, Tram HPB, Makram OM, Abdalla AS, Singh T, Hung I-C, et al., "Identifying SARS-CoV2 Transmission Cluster Category: An Analysis of Country Government Database," *Journal of Infection and Public Health* 14, no. 4 (2021): 461–467, https://doi.org/10.1016/j.jiph.2021.01.006.

20. Escandón et al., "COVID-19 False Dichotomies and a Comprehensive Review of the Evidence Regarding Public Health, COVID-19 Symptomatology, SARS-CoV-2 Transmission, Mask Wearing, and Reinfection"; CDC, "Choosing Safer Activities," May 28, 2021, https:// www.cdc.gov/coronavirus/2019-ncov/daily-life-coping/participate-in -activities.html; WHO, "Mask Use in the Context of COVID-19: Interim Guidance," December 1, 2020, https://apps.who.int/iris /handle/10665/337199; CDC, "Guidance for Wearing Masks," updated April 19, 2021, https://www.cdc.gov/coronavirus/2019-ncov/prevent -getting-sick/cloth-face-cover-guidance.html.

21. Escandón et al., "COVID-19 False Dichotomies and a Comprehensive Review of the Evidence Regarding Public Health, COVID-19 Symptomatology, SARS-CoV-2 Transmission, Mask Wearing, and Reinfection"; Slater SJ, Christiana RW, Gustat J, "Recommendations for Keeping Parks and Green Space Accessible for Mental and Physical Health During COVID-19 and Other Pandemics," *Preventing Chronic Disease* 17, no. E59 (2020): 200204, https://doi.org/10.5888/pcd17 .200204.

22. Mathai V, Das A, Bailey JA, Breuer K, "Airflows Inside Passenger Cars and Implications for Airborne Disease Transmission," *Science Advances* 7, no. 1 (2021): eabe0166, https://doi.org/10.1126/sciadv.abe0166; Allen JG, Ibrahim AM, "Indoor Air Changes and Potential Implications for SARS-CoV-2 Transmission," *Journal of the American Medical Association* 325, no. 20 (2021): 2112, https://doi.org/10.1001/jama.2021.5053; Halperin D, "A Marshall Plan for COVID-19," Real Clear Policy, November 5, 2020, https://www.realclearpolicy.com/articles/2020/11/05/a_marshall_plan_for_COVID-19_583019.html; WHO, "Roadmap to Improve and Ensure Good Indoor Ventilation in the Context of COVID-19," March 1, 2021, https://www.who.int/publications/i/item/9789240021280.

23. Escandón et al., "COVID-19 False Dichotomies and a Comprehensive Review of the Evidence Regarding Public Health, COVID-19 Symptomatology, SARS-CoV-2 Transmission, Mask Wearing, and Reinfection"; Halperin, "Coping with COVID-19: Learning from Past Pandemics to Avoid Pitfalls and Panic"; Hodgins S, Saad A, "Will the Higher-Income Country Blueprint for COVID-19 Work in Low- and Lower Middle-Income Countries?," *Global Health: Science and Practice* 8, no. 2 (2020): 136–143, https://doi.org/10.9745/GHSP-D-20-00217; Bavli I, Sutton B, Galea S, "Harms of Public Health Interventions Against COVID-19 Must Not Be Ignored," *BMJ* 371 (202): m4074, https://doi.org/10.1136/bmj.m4074.

24. Halperin, "Coping with COVID-19: Learning from Past Pandemics to Avoid Pitfalls and Panic"; CDC, "Guidance for Wearing Masks"; Bavli et al., "Harms of Public Health Interventions Against COVID-19 Must Not Be Ignored"; Douglas M, Katikireddi SV, Taulbut M, McKee M, McCartney G, "Mitigating the Wider Health Effects of COVID-19 Pandemic Response," *BMJ* 369 (2020): m1557, https://doi.org/10.1136/bmj.m1557; Ghosh R, Dubey MJ, Chatterjee S, Dubey S, "Impact of COVID-19 on Children: Special Focus on the Psychosocial Aspect," *Minerva Pediatrica* 72, no. 3 (2020): 226–235, https://doi.org/10.23736/S0026-4946.20.05887-9; Gunnell D, Appleby L, Arensman E, Hawton K, John A, Kapur N, et al., "Suicide Risk and Prevention During the COVID-19 Pandemic," *Lancet Psychiatry* 7, no. 6 (2020): 468–471, https://doi.org/10.1016/S2215-0366(20)30171-1; Marques ES, Moraes CL, Hasselmann MH, Deslandes SF, Reichenheim ME, "Violence Against Women, Children, and Adolescents During the COVID-19 Pandemic: Overview, Contributing Factors, and Mitigating Measures," *Cadernos de Saúde Pública* 36, no. 4 (2020): e00074420, https://doi

.org/10.1590/0102-311X00074420; Baral S, Rao A, Twahirwa Rwema JO, Lyons C, Cevik M, Kågesten AE, et al., "Competing Health Risks Associated with the COVID-19 Pandemic and Response: A Scoping Review," *medRxiv,* 2021, https://doi.org/10.1101/2021.01.07 .21249419; Chang AY, Cullen MR, Harrington RA, Barry M, "The Impact of Novel Coronavirus COVID-19 on Noncommunicable Disease Patients and Health Systems: A Review," *Journal of Internal Medicine* 289, no. 4 (2021): 450–462, https://doi.org/10.1111/joim.13184; Lin AL, Vittinghoff E, Olgin JE, Pletcher MJ, Marcus GM, "Body Weight Changes During Pandemic-Related Shelter-in-Place in a Longitudinal Cohort Study," *JAMA Network Open* 4, no. 3 (2021): e212536, https:// doi.org/10.1001/jamanetworkopen.2021.2536.

25.   Honein MA, Christie A, Rose DA, Brooks JT, Meaney-Delman D, Cohn A, et al., "Summary of Guidance for Public Health Strategies to Address High Levels of Community Transmission of SARS-CoV-2 and Related Deaths, December 2020," *Morbidity and Mortality Weekly Report* 69, no. 49 (2020): 1860–1867, https://doi.org/10.15585/mmwr.mm6949e2.

26.   Escandón et al., "COVID-19 False Dichotomies and a Comprehensive Review of the Evidence Regarding Public Health, COVID-19 Symptomatology, SARS-CoV-2 Transmission, Mask Wearing, and Reinfection."

27.   Bardsley M et al., "Epidemiology of Respiratory Syncytial Virus in Children Younger Than 5 Years in England During the COVID-19 Pandemic, Measured by Laboratory, Clinical, and Syndromic Surveillance: A Retrospective Observational Study," *Lancet Infectious Diseases* (September 2, 2022), https://www.sciencedirect.com/science /article/pii/S1473309922005254; Hartog GD, "Decline of RSV-Specific Antibodies During the COVID-19 Pandemic," *Lancet Infectious Diseases* (December 1, 2022), https://www.sciencedirect.com/science/article/pii /S1473309922007630; Baker RE, et al., "The Impact of COVID-19 Nonpharmaceutical Interventions on the Future Dynamics of Endemic Infections," *Proceedings of the National Academy of Sciences* 117, no. 48 (November 9, 2020), https://www.pnas.org/doi/full/10.1073/pnas .2013182117.

28.   Escandón et al., "COVID-19 False Dichotomies and a Comprehensive Review of the Evidence Regarding Public Health, COVID-19 Symptomatology, SARS-CoV-2 Transmission, Mask Wearing, and Reinfection"; Honein et al., "Summary of Guidance for Public Health Strategies to Address High Levels of Community Transmission of SARS-CoV-2 and Related Deaths, December 2020"; Escandón K, Martin

GP, Kuppalli K, Escandón K, "Appropriate Usage of Face Masks to Prevent SARS-CoV-2: Sharpening the Messaging amid the COVID-19 Pandemic," *Disaster Medicine and Public Health Preparedness* 15, no. 4 (2021): e5–e7, https://doi.org/10.1017/dmp.2020.336; Bo Y, Guo C, Lin C, Zeng Y, Li HB, Zhang Y, et al., "Effectiveness of Non-Pharmaceutical Interventions on COVID-19 Transmission in 190 Countries from 23 January to 13 April 2020," *International Journal of Infectious Diseases* 102 (2021): 247–253, https://doi.org/10.1016/j.ijid.2020.10.066; Haug N, Geyrhofer L, Londei A, Dervic E, Desvars-Larrive A, Loreto V, et al., "Ranking the Effectiveness of Worldwide COVID-19 Government Interventions," *Nature Human Behavior* 4, no. 12 (2020): 1303–1312, https://doi.org/10.1038/s41562-020-01009-0; Rasmussen AL, Escandón K, Popescu SV, "Facial Masking for COVID-19," *New England Journal of Medicine* 383, no. 21 (2020): 2092, https://doi.org/10.1056/NEJM c2030886.

29. Mondelli MU, Colaneri M, Seminari EM, Baldanti F, Bruno R, "Low Risk of SARS-CoV-2 Transmission by Fomites in Real-Life Conditions," *Lancet Infectious Diseases* 3099, no. 20 (2020): 30678, https://doi.org /10.1016/S1473-3099(20)30678-2; Goldman E, "Exaggerated Risk of Transmission of COVID-19 by Fomites," *Lancet Infectious Diseases* 20, no. 8 (2020): 892–893, https://doi.org/10.1016/S1473-3099(20)30561 -2; Meyerowitz EA, Richterman A, Gandhi RT, Sax PE, "Transmission of SARS-CoV-2: A Review of Viral, Host, and Environmental Factors," *Annals of Internal Medicine* 174, no. 1 (2021): 69–79, https://doi.org/10 .7326/M20-5008; Lewis D, "COVID-19 Rarely Spreads Through Surfaces. So Why Are We Still Deep Cleaning?," *Nature* 590, no. 7844 (2021): 26–28, https://doi.org/10.1038/d41586-021-00251-4; CDC, "Scientific Brief: SARS-CoV-2 Transmission," updated May 7, 2021, https://www.cdc.gov/coronavirus/2019-ncov/science/science-briefs/sars -cov-2-transmission.html.

30. Halperin DT, *Facing COVID Without Panic: 12 Common Myths and 12 Lesser Known Facts About the Pandemic, Clearly Explained by an Epidemiologist* (n.p.: Daniel Halperin, 2020); Thompson D, "Hygiene Theater Is Still a Huge Waste of Time," *The Atlantic,* February 8, 2021, https://www.theatlantic.com/ideas/archive/2021/02/hygiene-theater -still-waste/617939/; Yip L, Bixler D, Brooks DE, Clarke KR, Datta SD, Dudley S, et al., "Serious Adverse Health Events, Including Death, Associated with Ingesting Alcohol-Based Hand Sanitizers Containing Methanol—Arizona and New Mexico, May–June 2020," *Morbidity*

and Mortality Weekly Report 69, no. 32 (2020): 1070–1073, https://doi
.org/10.15585/mmwr.mm6932e1; Gharpure R, Hunter CM, Schnall
AH, Barrett CE, Kirby AE, Kunz J, et al., "Knowledge and Practices
Regarding Safe Household Cleaning and Disinfection for COVID-19
Prevention—United States, May 2020," *Morbidity and Mortality Weekly
Report* 69, no. 23 (2020): 705–709, https://doi.org/10.15585/mmwr
.mm6923e2; Chang A, Schnall AH, Law R, Bronstein AC, Marraffa
JM, Spiller HA, et al., "Cleaning and Disinfectant Chemical Exposures
and Temporal Associations with COVID-19—National Poison Data
System, United States, January 1, 2020–March 31, 2020," *Morbidity and
Mortality Weekly Report* 69, no. 16 (2020): 496–498, https://doi.org
/10.15585/mmwr.mm6916e1.

31. Lewis, "COVID-19 Rarely Spreads Through Surfaces. So Why Are We
Still Deep Cleaning?"; Halperin, *Facing COVID Without Panic.*

32. Rezasoltani S, Yadegar A, Hatami B, Asadzadeh Aghdaei H, Zali MR,
"Antimicrobial Resistance as a Hidden Menace Lurking Behind the
COVID-19 Outbreak: The Global Impacts of Too Much Hygiene on
AMR," *Frontiers in Microbiology* 11 (2020): 1–7, https://doi.org/10.3389
/fmicb.2020.590683; Makary M, Das I, Hashim F, Walsh C, "The Next
Pandemic Is Already Here," *MedPage Today,* January 20, 2021, https://
www.medpagetoday.com/blogs/marty-makary/90795.

33. Zhang XS, Duchaine C, "SARS-CoV-2 and Health Care Worker
Protection in Low-Risk Settings: A Review of Modes of Transmission
and a Novel Airborne Model Involving Inhalable Particles," *Clinical
Microbiology Reviews* 34, no. 2 (2020): e00009–21, https://doi.org/10
.1128/CMR.00184-20; Leung NHL, "Transmissibility and Transmission
of Respiratory Viruses," *Nature Reviews Microbiology* 19 (2021): 528–545,
https://doi.org/10.1038/s41579-021-00535-6.

34. Wright WF, Mackowiak PA, "Why Temperature Screening for
Coronavirus Disease 2019 with Noncontact Infrared Thermometers
Does Not Work," *Open Forum Infectious Diseases* 8, no. 1 (2021): 4–6,
https://doi.org/10.1093/ofid/ofaa603; Aw J, "The Non-Contact Handheld
Cutaneous Infra-Red Thermometer for Fever Screening During the
COVID-19 Global Emergency," *Journal of Hospital Infection* 104, no. 4
(2020): 451, https://doi.org/10.1016/j.jhin.2020.02.010; Dzien C, Halder
W, Winner H, Lechleitner M, "COVID-19 Screening: Are Forehead
Temperature Measurements During Cold Outdoor Temperatures Really
Helpful?," *Wiener klinische Wochenschrift* 133 (2021): 331–335, https://
doi.org/10.1007/s00508-020-01754-2; Normile D, "Airport Screening Is

Largely Futile, Research Shows," *Science* 367, no. 6483 (2020): 1177–1178, https://doi.org/10.1126/science.367.6483.1177; Kojima N, Klausner J, "It's Time to Ditch COVID-19 Temperature Checks," *Daily Beast,* May 14, 2021, https://www.thedailybeast.com/its-time-to-ditch-COVID-19-temperature-checks.

35. Mouchtouri V, Christoforidou E, an der Heiden L, Lemos CM, Fanos M, Rexroth U, Grote U, Belfroid E, Swaan C, Hadjichristodoulou C, "Exit and Entry Screening Practices for Infectious Diseases Among Travelers at Points of Entry: Looking for Evidence on Public Health Impact," *International Journal of Environmental Research and Public Health* 16, no. 23 (2019): 4638, https://doi.org/10.3390/ijerph16234638.

36. Mouchtouri VA, Bogogiannidou Z, Dirksen-Fischer M, Tsiodras S, Hadjichristodoulou C, "Detection of Imported COVID-19 Cases Worldwide: Early Assessment of Airport Entry Screening, 24 January Until 17 February 2020," *Tropical Medicine and Health* 48, no. 1 (2020): 79, https://doi.org/10.1186/s41182-020-00260-5.

37. Sette A, Crotty S, "Adaptive Immunity to SARS-CoV-2 and COVID-19," *Cell* 184, no. 4 (2021): 861–880, https://doi.org/10.1016/j.cell.2021.01.007.

38. Grubaugh ND, Hodcroft EB, Fauver JR, Phelan AL, Cevik M, "Public Health Actions to Control New SARS-CoV-2 Variants," *Cell* 184, no. 5 (2021): 1127–1132, https://doi.org/10.1016/j.cell.2021.01.044; Devi S, "Travel Restrictions Hampering COVID-19 Response," *Lancet* 395, no. 10233 (2020): 1331–1332, https://doi.org/10.1016/S0140-6736(20)30967-3.

39. Escandón et al., "COVID-19 False Dichotomies and a Comprehensive Review of the Evidence Regarding Public Health, COVID-19 Symptomatology, SARS-CoV-2 Transmission, Mask Wearing, and Reinfection"; Grubaugh et al., "Public Health Actions to Control New SARS-CoV-2 Variants"; Baker MG, Wilson N, Blakely T, "Elimination Could Be the Optimal Response Strategy for COVID-19 and Other Emerging Pandemic Diseases," *BMJ* 371 (2020): m4907, https://doi.org/10.1136/bmj.m4907.

40. Normile, "Airport Screening Is Largely Futile, Research Shows."

41. Grubaugh et al., "Public Health Actions to Control New SARS-CoV-2 Variants."

42. Binnicker MJ, "Challenges and Controversies to Testing for COVID-19," *Journal of Clinical Microbiology* 58, no. 11 (2020): e01695–20, https://doi.org/10.1128/JCM.01695-20.

43. Mina MJ, Andersen KG, "COVID-19 Testing: One Size Does Not Fit All," *Science* 371, no. 6525 (2021): 126–127, https://doi.org/10.1126/science.abe9187.

44. Cevik M, Tate M, Lloyd O, Maraolo AE, Schafers J, Ho A, "SARS-CoV-2, SARS-CoV, and MERS-CoV Viral Load Dynamics, Duration of Viral Shedding, and Infectiousness: A Systematic Review and Meta-Analysis," *Lancet Microbe* 2, no. 1 (2021): e13–e22, https://doi.org/10.1016/S2666-5247(20)30172-5; Walsh KA, Jordan K, Clyne B, Rohde D, Drummond L, Byrne P, et al., "SARS-CoV-2 Detection, Viral Load and Infectivity over the Course of an Infection," *Journal of Infection* 81, no. 3 (2020): 357–371, https://doi.org/10.1016/j.jinf.2020.06.067; Jefferson T, Spencer EA, Brassey J, Heneghan C, "Viral Cultures for COVID-19 Infectious Potential Assessment—A Systematic Review," *Clinical Infectious Diseases* 73, no. 11 (2021): e3884–e3889, https://doi.org/10.1093/cid/ciaa1764.

45. Levine-Tiefenbrun M, Yelin I, Katz R, Herzel E, Golan Z, Schreiber L, et al., "Initial Report of Decreased SARS-CoV-2 Viral Load After Inoculation with the BNT162b2 Vaccine," *Nature Medicine* 27 (2021): 790–792, https://doi.org/10.1038/s41591-021-01316-7; Petter E, Mor O, Zuckerman N, Oz-Levi D, Younger A, Aran D, et al., "Initial Real World Evidence for Lower Viral Load of Individuals Who Have Been Vaccinated by BNT162b2," *medRxiv*, February 8, 2021, https://doi.org/10.1101/2021.02.08.21251329; McEllistrem MC, Clancy CJ, Buehrle DJ, Lucas A, Decker BK, "Single Dose of a mRNA SARS-CoV-2 Vaccine Is Associated with Lower Nasopharyngeal Viral Load Among Nursing Home Residents with Asymptomatic COVID-19," *Clinical Infectious Diseases* 73, no. 6 (2021): e1365–e1367, https://doi.org/10.1093/cid/ciab263; CDC, "COVID-19 Interim Public Health Recommendations for Fully Vaccinated People," updated May 28, 2021, https://www.cdc.gov/coronavirus/2019-ncov/vaccines/fully-vaccinated-guidance.html.

46. Fillmore N, La J, Zheng C, Doron S, Do N, Monach P, et al., "The COVID-19 Hospitalization Metric in the Pre- and Post-Vaccination Eras as a Measure of Pandemic Severity: A Retrospective, Nationwide Cohort Study," Research Square, 2021, https://doi.org/10.21203/rs.3.rs-898254/v1; Denzer O, Nienaber M, "Germany Drops Incidence Levels as Key COVID Yardstick," Reuters, August 23, 2021, https://www.reuters.com/world/europe/german-drop-incidence-levels-key-COVID-yardstick-sources-2021-08-23/.

47. Bugin K, Woodcock J, "Trends in COVID-19 Therapeutic Clinical Trials," *Nature Reviews Drug Discovery* 20, no. 4 (2021): 254–255, https://doi.org/10.1038/d41573-021-00037-3.

48. Bedford J, Farrar J, Ihekweazu C, Kang G, Koopmans M, Nkengasong J, "A New Twenty-First Century Science for Effective Epidemic Response," *Nature* 575, no. 7781 (2019): 130–136, https://doi.org/10.1038/s41586-019-1717-y; Alam U, Nabyonga-Orem J, Mohammed A, Malac DR, Nkengasong JN, Moeti MR, "Redesigning Health Systems for Global Heath Security," *Lancet Global Health* 9, no. 4 (2021): e393–e394, https://doi.org/10.1016/S2214-109X(20)30545-3.

49. Escandón et al., "COVID-19 False Dichotomies and a Comprehensive Review of the Evidence Regarding Public Health, COVID-19 Symptomatology, SARS-CoV-2 Transmission, Mask Wearing, and Reinfection."